W0043339

DRUG THERAPY FOR TYPE 2 DIABETES

An Adis Pocket Reference

DRUG THERAPY FOR TYPE 2 DIABETES

An Adis Pocket Reference

Andrew J. Krentz MD, FRCP
Bedfordshire & Hertfordshire
Postgraduate Medical School,
United Kingdom

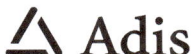 Adis

Editor: Louisa Mott
Design: Dan Benton
Copyeditor: Viv Lillywhite
Typesetter: MPS Limited. A Macmillan Company, Bangalore, India
Printer: Henry Ling Ltd, Dorchester, UK

Printed in the UK

ISBN 13: 978-1-908517-64-7

Copyright © Springer International Publishing Switzerland 2012. All Rights Reserved.

Springer Healthcare   Springer Science & Business Media UK Ltd
236 Gray's Inn Road   Chowley Oak Lane
London   Tattenhall, Chester
WC1X 8HB   CH3 9GA, UK

All rights reserved. This book is protected by copyright. No part of this book may be reproduced or transmitted in any form or by any means, including as photocopies or scanned-in or other electronic copies, or utilized by any information storage and retrieval system without written permission from the copyright owner, except for brief quotations embodied in critical articles and reviews. To request permission please contact: neil.scallion@springer.com.

DISCLAIMER

Care has been taken to confirm the accuracy of the information present and to describe generally accepted practices. However, the authors, editors, and publisher are not responsible for errors or omissions or for any consequences from application of the information in this book and make no warranty, expressed or implied, with respect to the currency, completeness, or accuracy of the contents of the publication. Application of this information in a particular situation remains the professional responsibility of the practitioner; the clinical treatments described and recommended may not be considered absolute and universal recommendations.

The authors, editors and publisher have exerted every effort to ensure that drug selection and dosage set forth in this text are in accordance with current recommendations and practice at the time of publication. However, in view of ongoing research, changes in government regulations, and the constant flow of information relating to drug therapy and drug reactions, the reader is urged to check the package insert for each drug for any change in indications and dosage and for added warnings and precautions. This is particularly important when the recommended agent is a new or infrequently employed drug.

Visit www.AdisOnline.com

CONTENTS

Dedicated to my family

Preface

This book aims to provide an update on drugs available for the treatment of type 2 diabetes and where they fit within current treatment algorithms.

The limited efficacy and tolerability of older drugs has spurred the development of several new classes of oral and injectable glucose-lowering agents with novel modes of action. These advances reflect progress in our understanding of the pathophysiology of type 2 diabetes. Old and newer drugs are increasingly being used side-by-side.

Type 2 diabetes is a highly complex and heterogeneous disorder that demands careful consideration of the risk-to-benefit profile of glucose-lowering drugs. The need for drug treatment to be tailored to the individual patient is a recurring theme throughout the text. The potential for serious unwanted effects, notably recent safety concerns about the risk of cardiovascular events, has led to more intense scrutiny of new agents. These risks have to be balanced against hopes for more effective long-term metabolic control, improved tolerability and better clinical outcomes. The higher cost of new drugs compared with long-established options is an important additional consideration for healthcare systems with finite resources.

Readers are directed to their national clinical guidance on use of these new drugs. It should be noted that the product licenses for individual agents not infrequently differ between countries. New indications and fixed-dose combinations can be expected to appear. Safety warnings from regulatory authorities should be heeded.

Andrew J. Krentz MD, FRCP
October 2012

Acknowledgements

Thanks go to the many colleagues that I have had the pleasure of collaborating with over the years. I thank Diabetes UK for their constructive comments on the manuscript. I am grateful to Louisa Mott and her colleagues at Springer Healthcare for their professionalism and forbearance.

Chapter 1

Type 2 diabetes: rationale for pharmacological treatment

1. Introduction

It is estimated that there are nearly 350 million adults with diabetes. Type 2 diabetes accounts for over 90% of this burden. The International Diabetes Federation (IDF) estimates that diabetes resulted in almost 4 million deaths in 2007. The World Health Organization (WHO) estimates that the number of people affected worldwide will grow to more than 470 million by 2030, the majority in low to middle-income countries. A powerful dose association exists between obesity and the risk of developing type 2 diabetes (Figure 1.1). The WHO estimates that more than 1 billion adults are over their ideal body weight, at least 300 million of them being clinically obese. The prevention of type 2 diabetes is a pressing public health issue. Translating the results of studies that have shown that intensive lifestyle measures i.e. weight reduction and increased levels of physical activity, can avert or postpone progression to diabetes is a formidable challenge.

Diabetes UK (www.diabetes.org.uk) calculates that the proportion of the UK population with diagnosed diabetes is over 4%, i.e. approximately 3 million people, the prevalence showing a strong association with increasing age. Another 850,000 or more may have as yet undiagnosed type 2 diabetes; this relects the often insidious nature of the development of type 2

Figure 1.1. Association between body mass index and risk of type 2 diabetes.

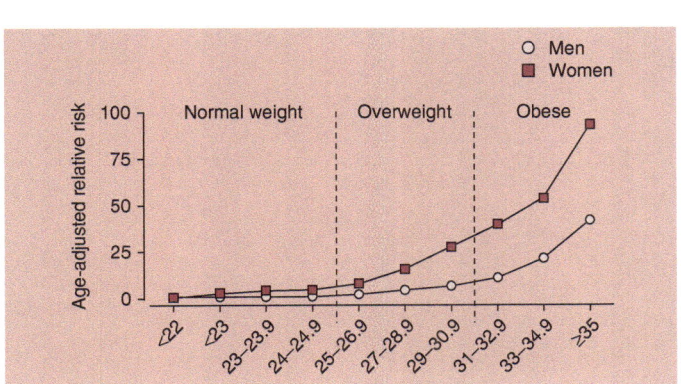

Adapted from Chan et al. (1994) and Colditz et al. (1995).

A. J. Krentz, *Drug Therapy for Type 2 Diabetes*,
DOI: 10.1007/978-1-908517-77-7_1,
© Springer International Publishing Switzerland 2012

diabetes with many years of pre-clinical disease. Casting the net wider, the number of people in the UK with less marked degrees of impaired glucose regulation is several fold higher. The adverse metabolic impact of excess adipose tissue is further modulated by anatomical patterns of fat accumulation, central or upper body adiposity being most dis-advantageous. The great majority of people with type 2 diabetes fall into the categories of overweight or obesity. Type 2 diabetes develops at a younger age in many non-white ethnic populations, and generally at lower levels of adiposity. The increasing prevalence of type 2 diabetes in obese adolescents and children is causing particular alarm. Studies suggest a high propensity to serious complications, such as progressive renal disease and coronary heart disease in individuals with early-onset type 2 diabetes.

A brief review of the presentation and diagnosis of type 2 diabetes is presented in Box 1.1 and Box 1.2.

1.1 Morbidity and premature mortality

Estimates of the global direct and indirect costs run to hundreds of billions of dollars. The largest component of direct costs is incurred from inpatient care, much of which reflects the burden of long-term microvascular and macrovascular complications. Occlusive atherothrombotic disease accounts

Box 1.1: Presentation and outline of diagnosis of type 2 diabetes

Type 2 diabetes may present with the classic symptoms of hyperglycaemia, i.e. thirst, polyuria, blurred vision, recurrent mucocutaneous infections, genital itching, slow wound healing and fatigue. These symptoms are, however, often inconspicuous. Type 2 diabetes frequently remains undiagnosed for ten years or more before it is identified during investigation of obesity, as part of a life insurance examination, cardiovascular risk assessment or following a serious vascular event. Presentation with advanced microvascular complications is uncommon, but subclinical or clinical vascular damage is often present at diagnosis. By the time they are diagnosed, half of the people with type 2 diabetes show signs of complications. Briefly, diagnosis rests on reliable (i.e. by laboratory) measurement of blood glucose, repeated if necessary particularly if the value is borderline or the patient is asymptomatic. A recent advance is the use of glycated haemoglobin to diagnose diabetes. Prominent osmotic symptoms, especially when accompanied by recent unintentional weight loss or ketonuria, point to marked insulin deficiency that warrants consideration of early insulin therapy. Even in the absence of ketonuria, any response to oral glucose-lowering agents is likely to be inadequate as a result of pronounced insulin deficiency. The situation can be more complex in non-white populations in whom ketosis may be transient. Hyperglycaemic emergencies, i.e. hyperosmolar non-ketotic hyperglycaemia and diabetic ketoacidosis are uncommon presentations.

Box 1.2: International Diabetes Federation standard care guidelines for diagnosis of type 2 diabetes

- *Each health service should decide whether to have a programme to detect people with undiagnosed diabetes. This decision should be based on the prevalence of undiagnosed diabetes and on the resources available to conduct the detection programme and treat those who are detected.*
- *Universal screening for undiagnosed diabetes is not recommended.*
- *Detection programmes should target high-risk people identified by an assessment of risk factors.*
- *Detection programmes should use the measurement of plasma glucose, preferably fasting. Individuals should have a repeat fasting plasma glucose measurement or HbA_{1c} followed by an oral glucose tolerance test to assess glycaemia.*
- *For diagnosis, an oral glucose tolerance test should be performed in people with a fasting plasma glucose of 5.6 mmol/l or greater and less than 7.0 mmol/l.*
- *When a random plasma glucose level of 5.6 mmol/l or greater and less than 11.1 mmol/l is detected on opportunistic screening, it should be repeated fasting, or an oral glucose tolerance test should be performed.*
- *Diabetes should not be diagnosed on the basis of a single laboratory measurement in the absence of symptoms.*
- *People with screen-detected diabetes should be offered treatment and care.*

Note: In 2010 the American Diabetes Association officially endorsed the diagnosis of diabetes using HbA_{1c} measurements (www.diabetes.org).

---

for approximately 70–80% of deaths among patients with type 2 diabetes. Coronary heart disease heads the list of causes of premature death, the risk being approximately two to fourfold higher in people with diabetes. While there is some evidence that life expectancy has improved in recent years diabetes continues to be associated with poorer clinical outcomes. Mortality after myocardial infarction is approximately threefold higher in the presence of diabetes. Type 2 diabetes is now the leading cause of end-stage renal failure, placing strains on renal replacement services; nephropathy further raises the risk of macrovascular disease and premature death. Retinopathy, neuropathy and foot complications cause considerable chronic disability.

1.2 Economic considerations

In the UK, it has been estimated that approximately 10% of the National Health Service (NHS) budget is accounted for by diabetes, some

£10 billion per annum; this figure seems certain to rise. The proportion spent on pharmacotherapy is relatively small; approximately 80% of the costs are incurred treating complications which theoretically could largely be avoided by excellent long-term metabolic control. Newer drugs are less likely to be widely available in countries with less well-developed economies; their cost may be many fold higher than older agents, especially those available as generic versions. Even in developed nations such as the UK the financial impact of new drugs is now carefully, if imprecisely, considered.

Less easily defined and quantified are the costs attributable to chronic disability, reflected by sick leave days or disability support payments. Neuropathy and recurrent foot ulceration, retinopathy and nephropathy often occur together. Diabetes has an appreciable, perhaps underestimated, negative impact on quality of life; patients tend to have lower scores in a range of assessments of general and mental health, particularly in the presence of major vascular complications.

1.3 The importance of metabolic control

Evidence from interventional clinical trials supports the contention that, when achieved safely (see Section 4 below), glycaemic control offers significant protection against the vascular and neurological complications of

Figure 1.2. UKPDS: Association between glycated haemoglobin (HbA$_{1c}$) and vascular complications.

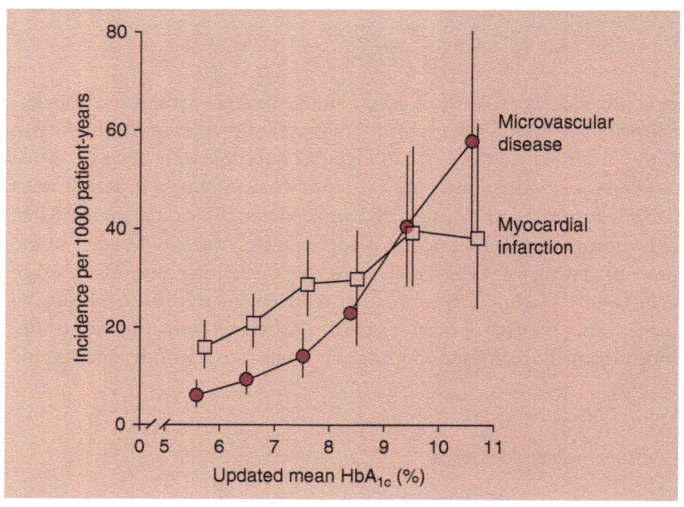

Data from: UK Prospective Diabetes Study (UKPDS 35) (2000), with permission.

Figure 1.3. UKPDS: Glycaemic control with monotherapy worsens over time.
A progressive rise in glycated haemoglobin (HbA$_{1c}$) occurred in groups receiving
conventional treatment, i.e. diet, and intensified treatment with sulphonylureas –
chlorpropamide and glibenclamide – and insulin.

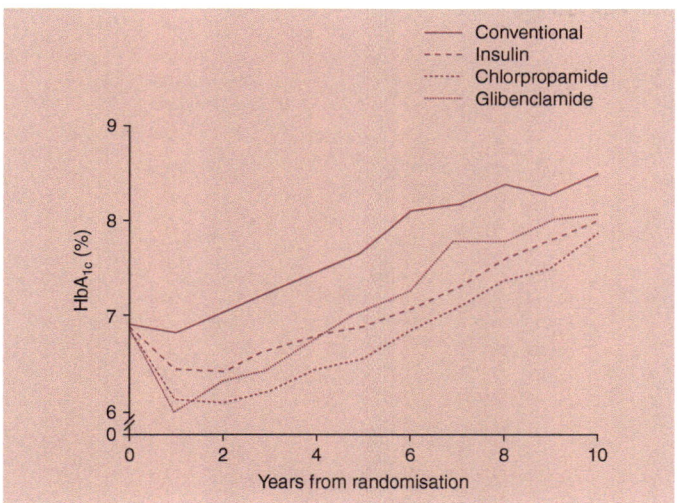

Data from: UK Prospective Diabetes Study (UKPDS 33) (1998a) and Wallace and Matthews (2003).

diabetes (Figure 1.2). This evidence is especially strong for retinopathy and
nephropathy. Appropriate strategies in selected groups also afford protection against macrovascular disease and can reduce mortality. Attaining and
sustaining good metabolic control soon after diagnosis is a key objective for
the majority of patients. This must be set within a policy of the systematic
identification and treatment of other modifiable vascular risk factors. It
should be appreciated at the outset that long-term normalisation of glucose
metabolism remains difficult to achieve (Figure 1.3) in large part because
of declining rates of insulin secretion (Figure 1.4). However, intensive
glycaemic control may not be suitable for all patients.

2. Type 2 diabetes: a progressive disorder

The progressive nature of type 2 diabetes was well illustrated by the
UKPDS (UK Prospective Diabetes Study), a randomised trial of 5102 newly
diagnosed type 2 patients followed for a median of 10 years while receiving
either conventional treatment, i.e. diet, or supplementary pharmacological

Figure 1.4. UKPDS: Islet β-cell function, assessed using modelling of fasting glucose and insulin concentrations, declines regardless of therapy in non-overweight and overweight patients treated with sulphonylureas or metformin (the latter only in an overweight subgroup). Note that β-cell function is only approximately 50% of normal at randomisation. There is a temporary improvement with sulphonylureas.

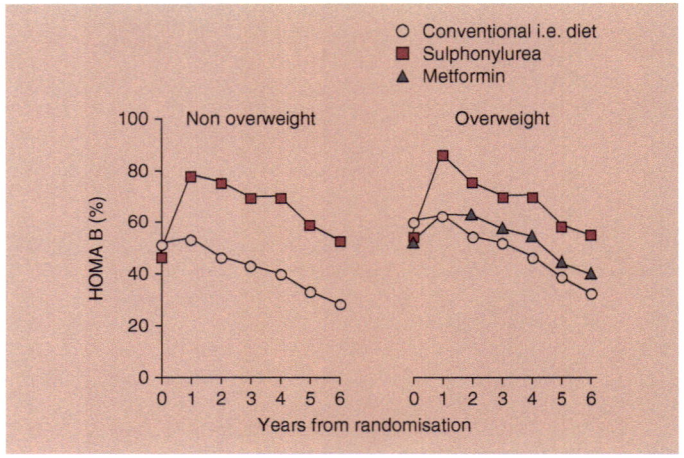

HOMA = Homeostasis model assessment.

Data from: UK Prospective Diabetes Study (UKPDS 16) (1995).

therapy with oral agents or insulin with the aim of comparing drugs from different classes. Insulin was started much earlier in the UKPDS than is usual in clinical practice as well as being used when the response to oral agents was deemed inadequate. Glycaemic control, which improved initially, deteriorated with time irrespective of the allocated treatment. This necessitated protocol amendments permitting drugs from other classes to be added as required.

2.1 UKPDS: Benefits of intensive glycaemic control

The improvement in glycaemic control afforded by intensive therapy [median glycated haemoglobin (HbA$_{1c}$) reduced by 0.9%] was associated with a 12% reduction in overall diabetes-related endpoints and a 25% (p = 0.0099) reduction in microvascular endpoints (Table 1.1A). The impact on myocardial infarction (16%) failed to attain statistical significance (p = 0.052). Overweight and obese patients assigned to metformin had significant reductions in macrovascular events, diabetes-related deaths and all-cause mortality compared with conventional therapy (Table 1.1B). These benefits did not appear to be related to the dose of metformin.

Taking the study population as a whole, further analysis showed that the benefits of intensive therapy continued to accrue as glucose levels were lowered into the non-diabetic range.

2.2 UKPDS: Post-trial follow-up study

The benefits of early glucose control were maintained during a 8.5-year post-trial follow-up during which glycaemic differences between the randomly assigned groups rapidly merged (Figure 1.5A). It has been suggested that this illustrates a glycaemic legacy effect, or metabolic memory, in which early intensive glycaemic control confers a longer-term reduction in vascular complications. In the sulphonylurea–insulin group, relative reductions in risk persisted for any diabetes-related endpoint (9%, p = 0.04) and microvascular disease (24%, p = 0.001). Risk reductions for myocardial infarction (15%, p = 0.01) and death from any cause (13%, p = 0.007) (Figure 1.5B) emerged as the number of events increased during the post-trial follow-up period. In the metformin treatment group, significant risk reductions persisted for any diabetes-related endpoint, myocardial infarction and death from any cause.

3. Pathophysiology

Appreciation of the pathophysiology of type 2 diabetes provides a framework within which to set behavioural and pharmacological interventions (Figure 1.6). Insights generated using ever more sophisticated research

Table 1.1. UK Prospective Diabetes Study (UKPDS) results.

		p value
A. Main results of intensive (sulphonylureas or insulin) versus conventional (diet) therapy[a]		
12%	Any diabetes-related endpoint	0.029
16%	Myocardial infarction	0.052
25%	Microvascular disease	0.0099
21%	Retinopathy at 12 years	0.015
33%	Albuminuria at 12 years	0.000054
B. Results of metformin versus conventional therapy in obese patients[b]		
32%	Any diabetes-related endpoint	0.002
39%	Myocardial infarction	0.01
30%	All macrovascular events	0.02
42%	Diabetes-related death	0.017
36%	All-cause mortality	0.011

[a]Data from: UKPDS 33 (1998a).
[b]Data from: UKPDS 34 (1998b).

Figure 1.5. UKPDS post-trial follow-up study. (A) The intensive and conventional treatment groups merge after the end of the randomised trial. (B) Emergence of significant reduction in all-cause mortality during the UKPDS post-trial follow-up study.

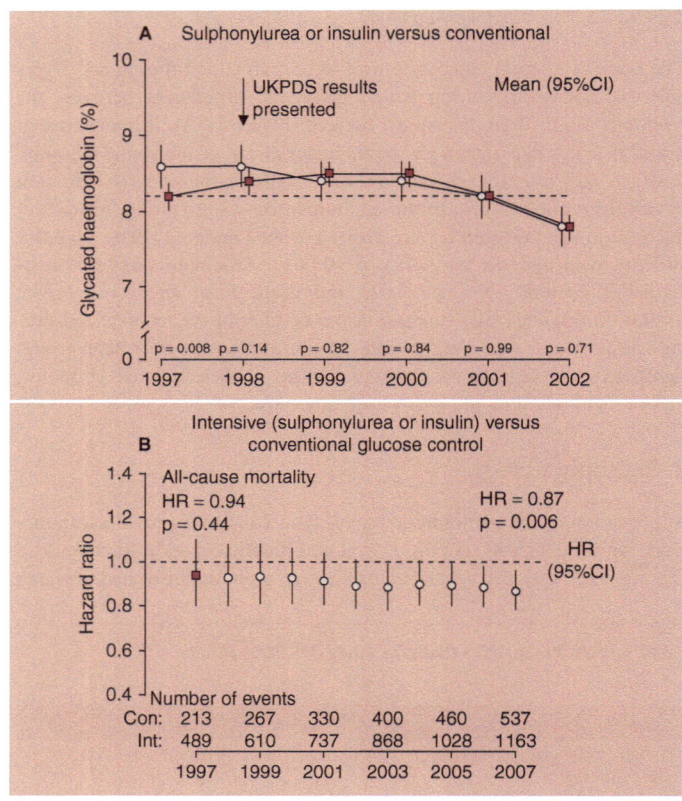

HR = Hazard ratio; UKPDS = UK Prospective Diabetes Study.

Data from: Holman et al. (2008), with permission from UKPDS.

techniques, however, provide only glimpses of the true complexity of type 2 diabetes. Add to this the interindividual heterogeneity that is readily apparent from daily clinical practice and the scene is set for what is a broad generalisation clouded by uncertainty. Genome-wide studies point to myriad mechanisms that may vary in terms of dose effect and differing combinations thereby accounting for some of the phenotypic variability of type 2 diabetes. To date, more than 40 susceptibiliy genes have been identified. These are further modified by ethnic, environmental, behavioural and nutritional influences. Pharmacogenetics – the study of genetic influences on response to drug therapy – is still in its infancy. Preliminary data suggest that certain gene variants may confer a better response to sulphonylureas or thiazolidinediones.

This matrix of interdependent genetic and environmental factors leads to defects in insulin secretion usually in the setting of impaired insulin action. Glucose tolerance does not become significantly impaired until the capacity of the islet β cells to compensate for defects in insulin action in target tissues reaches a critical threshold. Plasma insulin levels initially rise as glucose intolerance develops, but are insufficient to restore glucose levels to normal; eventually insulin secretion becomes deficient in absolute terms. Obesity, especially visceral adiposity, and abnormalities of glucagon secretion commonly contribute to impaired regulation of intermediary metabolism. Cellular metabolic disturbances in glucose and lipid handling participate both as causes and consequences thereby creating a vicious cycle.

3.1 Liver, muscle and adipose tissue

Insulin resistance in hepatocytes results in excessive rates of hepatic glucose production, the principal determinant of fasting blood glucose concentrations; this relationship is linear. Hepatocyte insulin resistance is also

---

Figure 1.6. Mechanisms of action of glucose-lowering treatments for type 2 diabetes. Note that secondary effects of glucose lowering include improved insulin action and insulin secretion.

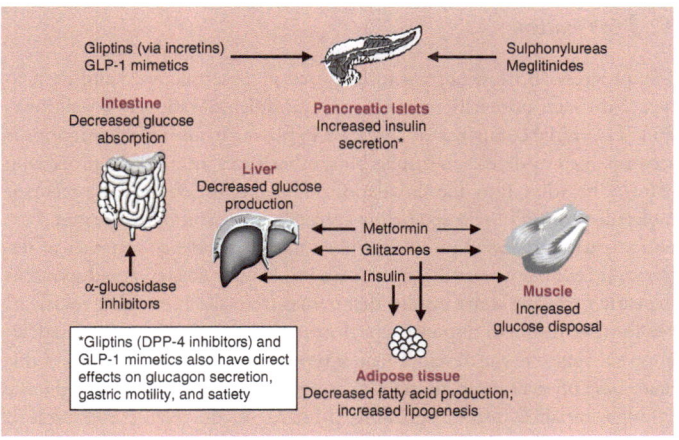

DPP-4 = Dipeptidyl peptidase 4; GLP-1 = glucagon-like peptide 1.

reflected in the impaired insulin-mediated suppression of hepatic glucose output after the ingestion of a meal.

Insulin resistance in muscle and adipose tissue impairs cellular glucose uptake. This reflects defects in insulin signalling resulting from inherent or acquired compromise of the complex cascade of events that follow the binding of insulin to its transmembrane receptor. The maximal effects of insulin in suppressing hepatic glucose production require lower concentrations than are needed to promote glucose disposal in skeletal muscle. Postprandial glucose intolerance thus tends to precede the appearance of appreciable fasting hyperglycaemia as insulin production wanes. In addition to genetic predisposition, insulin resistance in the liver and muscle result from the acquisition of obesity often compounded by insufficient physical activity. The antilipolytic effect of insulin is impaired in obesity and type 2 diabetes, resulting in elevated plasma concentrations of non-esterified fatty acids. These, in concert with fat-derived proinflammatory and proatherosclerotic cytokines, stimulate hepatic gluconeogenesis, promote insulin resistance and simultaneously reduce insulin secretion. Insulin sensitivity and impaired insulin secretion may also be exacerbated by hyperglycaemia *per se* – a phenomenon known as glucose toxicity. Enlarged fat cells have reduced lipid storage capacity. This may contribute to the deposition of fat in ectopic sites including the liver, muscle, pancreas and arteries. Lipid accumulation in the latter exacerbates insulin resistance, impairs insulin secretion and promotes atherosclerosis. The complexity of the relationship between obesity and glucose metabolism is further illustrated by evidence of impaired insulin signalling in the brain and the aforementioned defects in the regulation of fat-derived adipocytokines.

3.2 β-Cell function

The progression from normal to impaired glucose tolerance and then to type 2 diabetes primarily mirrors a profound deterioration in β-cell function. The initial compensatory increase in plasma insulin concentrations is accompanied by defects in insulin biosynthesis and intracellular processing before liberation into the circulation. The proportion of the precursor molecule proinsulin released before conversion to insulin is increased. Less potent partly processed proinsulin-like molecules serve as a marker of defective β cells before significant glucose intolerance ensues. A reduction in the early peak of plasma insulin that comes from the immediate release of pre-formed insulin in response to a glucose challenge is thought to mark an important stage in the development of type 2 diabetes. The blunting of this first phase of secretion is thought to contribute to a rise in plasma glucose through impaired insulin signalling, primarily in the liver. Restoration of first-phase insulin release is regarded as an important therapeutic objective when the emphasis is on the control of postprandial hyperglycaemia.

The continuing attrition of β cells, both in terms of individual and collective function, is accompanied by deposition of islet amyloid protein; this is accompanied by a reduction in β-cell mass. Insulin secretion occurs in tandem with the release of islet amyloid polypeptide in a 1:1 ratio. Islet amyloid polypeptide has the capacity to form toxic oligomers that have been implicated in β-cell dysfunction. Although the role of amyloid formation remains uncertain, the consequences of progressive losses of insulin-producing tissue are undisputed. A deleterious inflammatory process may accompany amyloid deposition.

Analysis of data from the UKPDS (Figure 1.4) suggests that by the time that type 2 diabetes is diagnosed β-cell function is already reduced by approximately 50%; in this trial no glucose-lowering drugs altered the loss of β-cell function, which approached 5% per annum. To date, no direct means of preventing this attrition has been reliably demonstrated, although some drugs may have a greater protective effect than others. The best that can be offered is a temporary and partial improvement by means of direct or indirect interventions that benefit the feedback between β cells and target tissues for insulin. These approaches underpin the use of glucose-lowering therapies for type 2 diabetes, up to the point that the loss of β-cell function necessitates insulin therapy. New treatment strategies using combinations of drugs that have shown some evidence suggesting preservation of β-cell function have yet to have their theoretical benefits confirmed in clinical trials.

3.3 The incretin system

Briefly, deficiency of intestinally-derived and glucose-stimulated glucagon-like peptide-1 (7–36) parallels the decline in β-cell function in type 2 diabetes. This hormone enhances the secretion of insulin in response to meals. Furthermore, β cells become resistant to the stimulatory effect of glucose-dependent insulinotropic polypeptide. Another action of glucagon-like peptide-1 is the suppression of glucagon secretion from islet α cells, thereby restraining a stimulatory effect on hepatic glucose production. The role of the incretin system in the pathogenesis of diabetes remains incompletely understood. The therapeutic implications of defects in the incretin axis are considered in more detail in Chapter 3.

4. Safety of intensive glucose-lowering strategies in high-risk patients

Post-UKPDS, data have been gathered from several large randomised trials that have tested the hypothesis that vascular complications are reduced through intensive glycaemic control. Although differing in study populations and methods, these studies share the common features that they: (a) moved beyond the glycaemic benchmark set by the UKPDS – i.e.

protection against macrovascular as well as microvascular complications, (b) were of less than 10 years' duration, and (c) recorded macrovascular event rates lower than anticipated. The latter observation points to changes in clinical practice with a move towards more comprehensive management of modifiable risk factors other than glucose in recent years. Of note, the UKPDS was performed in the pre-statin era, and when the importance of blood pressure was less well appreciated.

The results of the post-UKPDS glucose control trials have generated much discussion; for this reason they are considered in detail as they inform current clinical practice (Box 1.3).

Unexpectedly, the ACCORD (Action to Control Cardiovascular Risk in Diabetes) trial noted increased mortality during highly intensified (5% mortality, 257/5128 patients) compared with standard (4% mortality, 205/5123 patients) glycaemic management (Table 1.2). This may be ascribed to unique features of the trial design that lie outside customary clinical practice. The population, mean age 62 years, was at relatively high cardiovascular risk. The participants had a mean known duration of diabetes of 10 years. At entry to the study the median HbA_{1c} was 8.1%. In the intensive treatment group the aim was rapid achievement of a target HbA_{1c} of 6.0%. Extensive use of rosiglitazone and insulin, often together and in combination with sulphonylureas, may have contributed to high rates of hypoglycaemia and weight gain. The potential impact of hypoglycaemia on mortality in the ACCORD trial has been examined in post-hoc analyses. In both the intensive and conventional treatment groups one or more episodes of severe hypoglycaemia were associated with higher mortality compared with participants who had no hypoglycaemia. The risk of death associated with hypoglycaemia was, however, more pronounced among patients in the conventional treatment arm of the trial. Patients in the intensive treatment arm who did not achieve the glycaemic target also seemed to have a higher risk of mortality. These observations have been interpreted as evidence against hypoglycaemia explaining the increased relative risk of mortality in the intensive treatment group. It has been proposed that severe hypoglycaemia may be a marker for underlying factors, e.g. autonomic neuropathy, that could increase the risk of death. Older patients, those with lower body weight, or with renal impairment have been shown to be especially vulnerable to hypoglycaemia in clinical trials. Hypoglycaemia has long been considered to be potentially dangerous to the myocardium, and the contribution of hypoglycaemia to adverse outcomes in the ACCORD trial remains uncertain. Overall, lower HbA_{1c} levels were associated with lower mortality in patients assigned to either intensive or standard glucose control. A reduction in the primary outcome started to emerge after approximately 3 years in favour of the intensive treatment group. Subgroup analyses indicate that benefits of intensive therapy were evident in patients with no previous history of cardiovascular disease and those with lower HbA_{1c} concentrations at baseline.

Box 1.3: Summary of the main points of recent clinical trials that tested the hypothesis that intensive glycaemic control reduces macrovascular events in high-risk patients with type 2 diabetes

ACCORD (Action to Control Cardiovascular Risk in Diabetes): This was a large trial (10 251 participants) conducted in centres in the USA and Canada. While aiming to reduce cardiovascular events by intensive control (aiming for a glycated haemoglobin of <6.0%, but achieving a median of 6.4%) an unexpected increase in mortality was observed. Combinations of glucose-lowering drugs were used. These included sulphonylureas, often with insulin (in 77% of intensively treated patients at termination of the study) and rosiglitazone (92%). This strategy lowered glycated haemoglobin rapidly – over a few months – from a baseline median of 8.1%. The trial focused on relatively high-risk patients (mean age 62 years; known duration of diabetes 10 years), i.e. with a history of cardiovascular disease or additional risk factors. The trial was prematurely terminated (after 3.5 years) because of the aforementioned increased death rate in the intensive control arm. An increased frequency of severe hypoglycaemia and greater weight gain, more than 10 kg in almost 30% of the participants, was observed in the patients randomly assigned to intensified control. A 5-year follow-up study confirmed the earlier observation of an increased mortality signal in the intensive treatment group. In contrast, a reduction in the rate of myocardial infarction in this group was confirmed.

ADVANCE (Action in Diabetes and Vascular Disease: Preterax and Diamicron Modified Release Controlled Evaluation): This multinational study was the largest interventional clinical trial in type 2 diabetes with 11 140 participants, mean age 66 years and a mean duration of diabetes of 8 years. Good glycaemic control, as judged by glycated haemoglobin, was attained gradually over 36 months (from a baseline median of 7.2%) using a well-defined regimen based on once-daily diamicron MR (modified release gliclazide). The dose of diamicron MR was increased progressively to a maximum of 120 mg daily; agents from other classes were then added as required in a suggested sequence, the next set being metformin. Insulin, which was being used as additional therapy in 41% of intensively treated patients at the end of the study (after 5.0 years), was initiated as a once-daily dose of a basal preparation and intensified with additional injections if necessary. The use of thiazolidinediones was much lower than in the ACCORD trial. The target glycated haemoglobin concentration, a mean of 6.5%, was achieved and sustained until the end of the study, a median of 5 years. This represented a time-weighted average reduction of 0.67 percentage points compared with the standard therapy group. Intensified therapy reduced severe diabetic complications thanks to a significant 10% reduction on microvascular and macrovascular combined endpoints. At the microvascular level, the development and progression of renal microvascular complications, principally the appearance and progression of albuminuria were decreased, allied to increased rates of

Continued on next page

Box 1.3: Continued.

regression of albuminuria. At the macrovascular level, the strategy provides a trend towards a reduction in cardiovascular death. Importantly, there was no suggestion of harm and a suggestion of benefit; this contrasts with the results of the ACCORD trial. It is noteworthy that the ADVANCE trial, like ACCORD, selected participants with a relatively high predicted risk of macrovascular events. A higher incidence of major hypoglycaemia was encountered during intensified treatment, although at a lower rate than in the UKPDS, and in the context of better glycaemic control. Again, in contrast to the ACCORD trial, there was weight neutrality in the intensively treated group over the duration of the study.

VADT (Veterans Affairs Diabetes Trial): This study focused on a group of mainly male military veterans with a mean age of 60 years, known duration of diabetes 11.5 years, and the worst glycaemic control of any of the studies – a glycated haemoglobin level of 9.5% at baseline. The VADT study recruited patients at the highest predicted risk in any of the three trials. The achieved glycated haemoglobin levels were 6.9% and 8.4% in the intensive and standard therapy groups. As in the ACCORD trial, combinations of oral drugs, including glimepiride and rosiglitazone, in combination with insulin (in 90%) were employed in the intensive treatment arm. There was no impact of improved glycaemic control on microvascular or macrovascular complications over 7.5 years. No excess mortality was noted. Greater weight gain and a higher incidence of hypoglycaemia were observed with intensified therapy. Severe hypoglycaemia, defined as loss of consciousness or severe change in consciousness, was associated with an increased risk of cardiovascular events and in both the standard and intensive treatment groups.

Two other large trials of intensified glucose-lowering therapy, AD-VANCE (Action in Diabetes and Vascular Disease: Preterax and Diamicron Modified Release Controlled Evaluation) and the VADT (Veterans Affairs Diabetes Trial), did not show any excess risk of vascular events overall. In the VADT study, however, participants who experienced severe hypoglycaemia had a significantly higher risk of having a cardiovascular event in subsequent months.

ADVANCE – In this trial there was no evidence of an increased risk of cardiovascular events from intensive glucose control; significant reductions in the onset and progression of nephropathy were observed. The therapeutic strategy used in the ADVANCE trial provided a gradual reduction in HbA_{1c} using once-daily modified release gliclazide as foundation therapy, and adding other agents in sequence aiming for a target of 6.5%. This was achieved with a significantly lower rate of severe hypoglycaemia than that seen in the ACCORD trial and with minimal weight gain overall compared with standard therapy. A five year post-trial follow-up is now in progress.

VADT – This trial showed no overall evidence of cardiovascular benefits from improved glycaemic control; moreover, weight gain and hypogly-caemia were prominent consequences of intensified therapy. Of note, if diabetes had been diagnosed more than 20 years before intensive glucose control was initiated the risk of a cardiovascular event doubled. In patients within 15 years of diagnosis, intensive therapy reduced cardiovascular events including mortality. No protection was evident in patients within 15–20 years from diagnosis, and among patients with a longer known duration of diabetes, intensive therapy was associated with worse outcomes compared with standard therapy.

A series of meta-analyses sought to amalgamate data from the afore-mentioned trials along with data from some other relevant studies. This exercise provided some broad conclusions and generated recommenda-tions about the value of good glycaemic control in reducing cardiovascular events. Taking the three studies, along with UKPDS and the PROactive (PROspective PioglitAzone Clinical Trial in MacroVascular Events) trial,

Table 1.2. Major post-UKPDS clinical trials that have tested the hypothesis that intensive glycaemic control reduces cardiovascular disease.

Study	HbA$_{1c}$ %	Primary outcome	HR (95% CI) for primary outcome	HR (95% CI) for mortality
ACCORD (n = 10 250)	7.5 vs 6.4	Non-fatal MI, non-fatal stroke, CVD death	0.90 (0.78–1.04)	1.22 (1.01–1.46) p = 0.04
ADVANCE (n = 11 140)	7.3 vs 6.5	Non-fatal MI, non-fatal stroke, CVD death	0.94 (0.84–1.06)	0.93 (0.83–1.06)
VADT (n = 1700)	8.4 vs 6.9	MI, stroke, death from cardiovascular causes, new/ worsening CHF, revascularisation and inoperable CAD, amputation for ischaemic gangrene	0.87 (0.73–1.04)	1.06 (0.801–1.416)

ACCORD: Action to Control Cardiovascular Risk in Diabetes; ADVANCE: Action in Diabetes and Vascular Disease: Preterax and Diamicron Modified Release Controlled Evaluation; CAD: coronary artery disease; CHF: congestive heart failure; CVD: cardiovascular disease; HbA$_{1c}$: glycated haemoglobin; HR: hazard ratio; MI: myocardial infarction; UKPDS: UK Prospective Diabetes Study; VADT: Veterans Affairs Diabetes Trial. Glycated haemoglobin levels are those achieved for standard and intensive therapy groups at the end of the study.

> **Box 1.4: Summary of main clinical practice points from recent trials examining the influence of tight glycaemic control on cardiovascular events in patients with type 2 diabetes**
>
> - *Macrovascular risk reduction, limited to non-fatal myocardial infarction and other coronary events with no impact on stroke, was in line with estimates from observational studies, i.e. approximately 15%.*
> - *The impact of glucose control, in terms of numbers needed to treat, was lower than for blood pressure control or statin therapy.*
> - *No reduction, or increase, in cardiovascular or all-cause mortality, was observed in intensively treated patients.*
> - *Patients with no history of cardiovascular disease gained benefit from intensified control, whereas those with macrovascular complications did not.*
> - *There was no reduction in cardiovascular deaths over the relatively short time span of the studies.*
> - *The balance of risks and benefits may vary between different patient groups.*

the average overall difference in glycated haemoglobin between intensive and standard treatments was just under 1%, the ACCORD and VADT studies having the largest reductions. Key points from these meta-analyses are summarised in Box 1.4. Adding to the debate about glycaemic targets was a retrospective cohort study in patients with type 2 diabetes published in 2010, which reported a U-shaped association with the lowest death and lowest event rates seen at an HbA_{1c} level of 7.5%.

There is broad agreement among clinicians and expert groups that glucose-lowering regimens should be tailored to individual circumstances. The current data have been interpreted to suggest that in general a cautious approach to intensive glucose-lowering therapy should be exercised in higher-risk patients. Efforts should always be directed to minimising the risk of hypoglycaemia, especially in older patients and in individuals with cardiovascular disease. The ACCORD trial results suggest that patients free of cardiovascular disease might derive cardiovascular protection from intensive glycaemic control. The VADT study data implicate the known duration of type 2 diabetes as a modulating factor. The UKPDS follow-up study suggests that better glycaemic control in the years immediately after diagnosis may ultimately bring cardiovascular benefits over a longer time-scale. Many additional hypotheses have been generated by these recent studies that can only be tested in well-designed clinical trials. The availability of newer drugs that carry lower risks of hypoglycaemia and weight gain might alter the balance of risks and benefits of intensive glycaemic control. This remains a complex area of clinical practice with many unresolved issues.

4.1 Cardiovascular safety of new drugs

Phase III clinical trials aimed at achieving approval from regulatory authorities tend to focus on highly selected patients. Candidates with diabetes that is accompanied by advanced cardiac, renal, or hepatic disease tend to be excluded. Extrapolation of risks and benefits from these trials to the broader and more complex case mix encountered in daily practice can present many difficulties. Short-term trials early in the life cycle of a new drug may mean that evidence of harm comes to light only after years of clinical use. Greater caution from regulatory authorities has come in the wake of recent concerns about the cardiovascular safety of rosiglitazone. In 2008 the US Food and Drug Adminstration (FDA) issued guidance recommending that all new drugs developed for the treatment of type 2 diabetes be evaluated to ensure cardiovascular safety. The approval of some newer drugs for type 2 diabetes has been deferred pending further safety data. The European Medicines Agency (EMA) has also published safety requirements that new glucose-lowering drugs must satisfy. Safety concerns extend to weight-reducing drugs used in patients with diabetes; as discussed in Chapter 2, sibutramine was suspended from use in Europe early in 2010 in response to adverse clinical trial data. Also in 2010, the EMA issued its own draft guidance concerning the evaluation of cardiovascular safety of new diabetes drugs.

5. Therapeutic approaches

A dose–effect association between average glucose control and the risk of vascular complications has been demonstrated in several clinical trials. Adequate treatment of hyperglycaemia is thus an essential component of individualised care plans for patients with type 2 diabetes. This often represents a major challenge, not least because of the limited effectiveness and tolerability of behavioural and pharmacological interventions. The arrival of new drug classes that are weight-neutral or weight-reducing, and carry a negligible risk of hypoglycaemia, has prompted a reappraisal of traditional approaches to initiating and escalating glucose-lowering therapy. This debate is reflected in the differing recommendations between major expert committees and is discussed in more detail in Chapter 4. Differences in the impact of different drug classes on fasting versus postprandial glucose concentrations have not translated into clear clinical benefits. Therefore, established and newer agents are selected on criteria that include: perceived advantages and disadvantages; patient and physician preference; tolerability and safety profiles; and cost – to the patient directly or through insurance or government schemes.

5.1 Lifestyle measures

The management of type 2 diabetes hinges on lifestyle changes supplemented in most instances by glucose-lowering drugs. Access to education

Figure 1.7. Outline of therapeutic approach to the treatment of type 2 diabetes. Whereas different guidelines vary in timing, recommendations of specific drug use at each stage, and glycaemic thresholds for intervention at each stage, there is agreement that a step-wise escalation of glucose-lowering therapy is required as type 2 diabetes progresses.

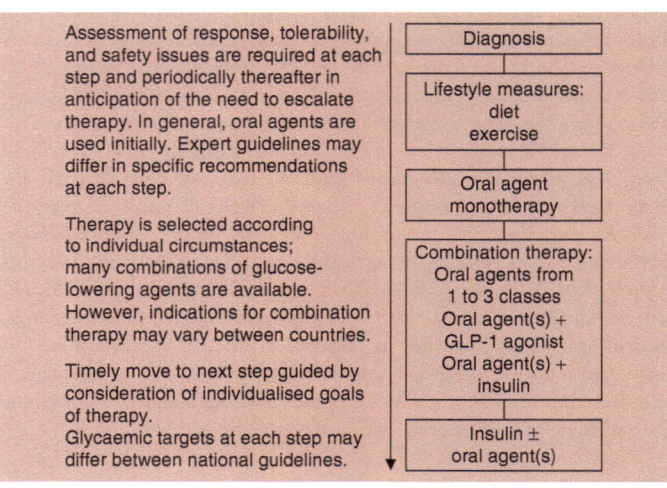

Assessment of response, tolerability, and safety issues are required at each step and periodically thereafter in anticipation of the need to escalate therapy. In general, oral agents are used initially. Expert guidelines may differ in specific recommendations at each step.

Therapy is selected according to individual circumstances; many combinations of glucose-lowering agents are available. However, indications for combination therapy may vary between countries.

Timely move to next step guided by consideration of individualised goals of therapy.
Glycaemic targets at each step may differ between national guidelines.

Diagnosis

Lifestyle measures: diet exercise

Oral agent monotherapy

Combination therapy: Oral agents from 1 to 3 classes Oral agent(s) + GLP-1 agonist Oral agent(s) + insulin

Insulin ± oral agent(s)

Arrow indicates deteriorating glycaemic control over time

GLP-1 = Glucagon-like peptide-1.

and professional multidisciplinary support – as well as drug therapy – shows considerable variations between countries. At best, partial restoration of metabolism is achieved in the great majority of patients; timely escalation of glucose-lowering therapy is required. This implies the step-wise use of combinations of agents from different classes. Insulin therapy is ultimately required in a large proportion of patients (Figure 1.7). For a minority of patients with osmotic symptoms or impending major metabolic decompensation insulin is required from the outset.

Currently, only bariatric surgery, available in the UK only for small numbers of highly selected patients, can consistently provide a convincing solution to obesity-associated type 2 diabetes. Associated vascular risk factors, including elevated blood pressure, dyslipidaemia and insulin resistance, are also improved. When present in combination, as they are in the majority of patients with type 2 diabetes, the risk of atherothrombotic events is heightened.

The management of type 2 diabetes must take into account co-morbidities, individual social circumstances, health literacy and cultural issues. In recent years, the model of care has moved away from a didactic approach to the empowerment of patients with the aim of engaging the patient in setting short and longer-term goals while striving to improve, or at least not to compromise quality of life. In the UK, multidisciplinary teams offer advice on lifestyle and diet, measures to address modifiable cardiovascular risk and the selection of realistic treatment targets. In the UK the introduction of financial incentives has been credited with driving some of the improvements in the process and attainment of treatment targets seen over the past few years. The primary care team has assumed responsibility for managing the majority of patients; specialist services are brought into play when additional expertise is required, e.g. diabetes during pregnancy, managing major complications such as progressive ne-phropathy. Ongoing support that is responsive to changing needs and circumstances is required. Periodic reviews focussed on identifying early complications, i.e. neuropathy, retinopathy and nephropathy, are mandatory. An assessment of cardiovascular risk is required, and appropriate measures instituted with respect to major modifiable risk factors. Self-management is the key to success. Patients must be equipped with the requisite knowledge and skills to manage their diabetes effectively.

The concepts of dietary modification, adequate levels of physical activity and other lifestyle measures should be introduced at diagnosis; this advice should be reinforced periodically. These measures can provide valuable blood glucose-lowering efficacy and may enable glycaemic targets to be achieved, at least in the short term. Intensive group education programmes such as DESMOND (Diabetes Education and Self-management for Ongoing and Newly Diagnosed) in the UK can produce reductions in glycated haemoglobin of approximately 1.5% at 12 months. Drug therapy should be introduced promptly if glycaemic targets are not met or not maintained. It is important to explain the high probability of requiring adjunctive pharmacological therapy so that patients do not feel that their efforts have been in vain. Continued engagement with lifestyle modifications may translate into useful reductions in the intensity of drug therapy.

6. Guidelines and treatment algorithms

Care should be taken to avoid the burden of treatment becoming disproportionate to the objectives of therapy. The inevitable need for polypharmacy brings problems of concordance, especially if therapy is not tolerated; all drugs used in the treatment of diabetes have the capacity to impair quality of life, cause serious harm, or in some cases be lethal if used inappropriately. The complex array of therapies, many of which can be used in combination, presents the non-specialist prescribing clinician with ever more complex challenges. Current treatment algorithms aim to provide a framework for initiating and intensifying glucose-lowering therapy. Some examples consider the economic impact of new therapies more overtly than others. Whichever is used, such algorithms should never replace good clinical judgement that is in line with the patient's needs and informed personal objectives.

6.1 Glycaemic targets

There are some variations in the glycaemic targets proposed by national and international expert groups. The American Diabetes Association (ADA) sets a general target for HbA_{1c} of less than 7.0%. This is qualified by the view that for some patients glycaemic control should be as close to normality as possible without causing significant hypoglycaemia. After considering the results of the ACCORD, ADVANCE and VADT studies a position statement was issued jointly in 2008 by the ADA, the American College of Cardiology (ACC) and the American Heart Association (AHA) recommending that in general the target should not be lowered below 7.0%. Moreover, for patients with a history of severe hypoglycaemia, limited life expectancy, advanced microvascular or macrovascular complications, extensive comorbid conditions, and those with longstanding diabetes in whom the treatment goals prove difficult to attain, less stringent goals should be considered.

The ADA/European Association for the Study of Diabetes (EASD) consensus guidelines propose that an HbA_{1c} of 7.0% or greater should prompt consideration of further action to reduce hyperglycaemia within the proposed algorithm. The aim is to achieve an HbA_{1c} of at least less than 7.0%, safe attainment of normal glucose levels being the ultimate goal. The American Association of Clinical Endocrinologists (AACE) and the IDF set their HbA_{1c} targets at less than 6.5% (Table 1.3). The caveats concerning individualised risk assessment with consideration of higher targets for vulnerable patients apply.

In England, Wales and Scotland primary care doctors receive remuneration partly based on achieving specified glycaemic targets for

Table 1.3. Glycaemic targets proposed by expert groups.

Organisation	HbA$_{1c}$ (%)	FPG (mmol/l)	PPG (mmol/l)
ADA/EASD	<7.0	–	–
IDF Europe	<6.5	5.5 (<100)[a]	7.8 (<140)[a]
AACE	≤6.5	6.1 (<110)[a]	7.8 (<140)[a]

[a]mg/dl.
AACE: American Association of Clinical Endocrinologists; ADA: American Diabetes Association; EASD: European Association for the Study of Diabetes; FPG: fasting plasma glucose; HbA$_{1c}$: glycated haemoglobin; IDF: International Diabetes Federation; PPG: postprandial glucose.

patients with diabetes. There is evidence that diabetes care has improved in recent years, coincident with the introduction of this approach.

The 2009 recommendations of the National Institute for Health and Clinical Excellence (NICE) for England and Wales recommend a general glycated haemoglobin of 6.5%; this is set at 7.5% for those at risk of severe hypoglycaemia. NICE reminds healthcare professionals that even these targets will not be achieved by everyone, nor are they appropriate for all patients. For patients treated with lifestyle measures alone or who are taking one drug, the recommended target HbA_{1c} is 6.5% (Diabetes Control and Complications Trial aligned) or 48 mmol/mol (International Federation of Clinical Chemistry and Laboratory Medicine standardised).[1] As recommended in other guidelines a target above this level might, however, be appropriate for some patients, a decision that should be made in the light of individual circumstances. For people taking two or more glucose-lowering agents, including insulin, the usual target HbA_{1c} is less than 7.5% (59 mmol/mol). A higher target may be deemed appropriate when the balance of risks, benefits and burden of therapy are considered. The use of highly intensive pharmacological strategies to achieve HbA_{1c} levels less than 6.5% (48 mmol/mol) rapidly should generally be avoided. Response to therapy should be individually assessed by the measurement of HbA_{1c} until stable control is achieved.

6.2 Choice of drug therapy: weighing benefits and risks

The main classes of oral glucose-lowering drugs and their principal modes of action are listed in Table 1.4. The efficacy of each class, together

---

[1]**Standardisation of HbA_{1c}:** The new standard for HbA_{1c} has been developed by the International Federation of Clinical Chemistry and Laboratory Medicine (IFCC). IFCC-standardised values of HbA_{1c} are expressed as mmol per mol of total haemoglobin (mmol/mol). From June 2011, results in the UK will be reported only in IFCC-standardised units.

Comparison of DCCT-aligned and IFCC-standardised HbA_{1c} values.

DCCT-aligned HbA_{1c} units (%)	IFCC-standardised HbA_{1c} units (mmol/mol)
6.0	42
6.5	48
7.0	53
7.5	59
8.0	64
9.0	75

DCCT: Diabetes Control and Complications Trial; IFCC: International Federation of Clinical Chemistry and Laboratory Medicine.

Table 1.4. Classes of oral glucose-lowering drugs and their main modes of action. Not all drugs listed are available in every country.

Class	Main mode of glucose lowering	Main cellular mechanism of action
Biguanide Metformin	Counter insulin resistance; decrease hepatic glucose output	Enhance a range of insulin-dependent and independent actions including AMPK activation

Sulphonylureas
  Glimepiride
  Gliclazide
  Glibenclamide
  (glyburide in USA)
  Glipizide
  Tolbutamide
  Chlorpropamide
	Stimulate insulin secretion for ~6–24 h	Bind to SUR-1 sulphonylurea receptors on islet β cells, which closes ATP-sensitive Kir6.2 potassium channels

Meglitinides
  Repaglinide
  Nateglinide
	Stimulate insulin secretion (faster onset and shorter duration of action than sulphonylureas)	Bind to benzamido site on SUR-1 receptors on pancreatic β cells, which closes ATP-sensitive Kir6.2 potassium channels

Gliptins (DPP-4 inhibitors)
  Sitagliptin
  Vildagliptin
  Saxagliptin
  Linagliptin
	Increase prandial insulin secretion; reduce glucagon secretion	Inhibit DPP-4 enzyme thereby increasing the plasma concentrations of insulinotropic incretin hormones

Thiazolidinediones (PPARγ agonists)
  Pioglitazone
  Rosiglitazone
	Increase insulin sensitivity, especially insulin-mediated glucose utilization	Activate nuclear receptor PPARγ mainly in adipose tissue, which affects insulin action and glucose–fatty acid cycle

α-Glucosidase inhibitors
  Acarbose
  Miglitol
  Voglibose
	Slow the rate of intestinal carbohydrate digestion	Competitive inhibition of intestinal α-glucosidase enzymes

AMPK: Adenosine 5′-monophosphate-activated protein kinase; ATP: adenosine triphosphate; DPP-4: dipeptidyl peptidase 4; PPARγ: peroxisome proliferator-activated receptor gamma; SUR-1: sulphonylurea receptor 1.

with main cautions and contraindications, are listed in Table 1.5. At each stage of treatment the best choice should be made based on an appreciation of the potential benefits and hazards of treatment for a given patient. The early initiation of glucose-lowering drugs and lower pre-treatment glycated

Table 1.5. Main features of oral glucose-lowering treatments for type 2 diabetes.

	Metformin	Sulphonylureas	Meglitinides	Thiazolidinediones	Gliptins	α-Glucosidase inhibitors
HbA₁c	↓ ~1–2%	↓ ~1–2%	↓ ~0.5–1.5%	↓ ~1–1.5%	↓ ~0.5–1.0%	↓ ~0.5–1%
Body weight	–/↓	↑	↑/–	↑	–	–
Lipids	–/+	–	–	+/–/×	–	–/+
Blood pressure	–	–	–	↓/–	–	–
Tolerability	Gastrointestinal	Hypoglycaemia	Hypoglycaemia	Fluid retention	–	Gastrointestinal
Safety issues	Lactic acidosis	Hypoglycaemia	Hypoglycaemia	Oedema Anaemia Heart failure Skeletal fractures Bladder cancer (pioglitazone)	–	–
Cautions	Renal function Liver function States of hypoxia	Liver function Renal function	Liver function Renal function	Cardiovascular disease Osteoporosis	Liver function (vildagliptin) Renal function (sitagliptin; vildagliptin. Reduce saxagliptin dose: not recommended in severe renal failure requiring dialysis)	Inflammatory bowel disease

HbA₁c: glycated haemoglobin; +: benefit; ↓: decreased; ×: impair; ↑: increased; –: neutral.
A caution mandates appropriate investigations prior to and during therapy. The latest prescribing information should be checked for each individual drug. This is especially important with respect to safety issues.

haemoglobin concentrations appear to be associated with better attainment and durability of glycaemic control. Specific objectives of therapy may be an additional consideration. For example, deciding whether to target fasting or postprandial hyperglycaemia – ideally both together – involves choices of agents and how they can best be combined. Appropriate monitoring is required to gauge response and titrate therapy. Factors such as race, gender, body weight and the presence of comorbidities should be borne in mind. It also needs to be appreciated that the evidence favouring one class of glucose-lowering drug over another in terms of impact on long-term clinical outcomes remains tenuous.

6.3 Additional considerations in subgroups of patients

Children and adolescents – The increasing prevalence of type 2 diabetes among the young adds an extra dimension to risk–benefit considerations. There is limited experience with oral glucose-lowering agents in these age groups; expert advice should be sought.

Women of childbearing age – When treating type 2 diabetes in women of childbearing age the risk of unplanned pregnancy while receiving drug therapy should always be borne in mind. The risks and benefits of glucose-lowering agents must be carefully considered. Insulin remains the preferred option for glucose control in pregnancy. For more detailed guidance see NICE clinical guideline 63 (2008). Metformin is extensively used off-licence in women with polycystic ovary syndrome.

The elderly – Older patients tend to be more vulnerable to most of the cautions and contraindications to glucose-lowering drugs. Unpredictable deteriorations in renal, hepatic or vascular function can occur rapidly, necessitating more frequent monitoring. These and other comorbidities are common. Hypoglycaemia is a particular concern in this age group, especially among the frail and those with cardiovascular disease. Moreover, symptomatic hypoglycaemia may be more difficult to diagnose in the elderly. Limited life expectancy and quality of life issues are often important considerations when setting glycaemic targets. The wishes of the patient and their relatives should inform these decisions. Further guidance is offered in the clinical guidelines of the European Diabetes Working Party for Older People, 2001-2004.

Further reading

Action to Control Cardiovascular Risk in Diabetes Study group. Effects of intensive glucose lowering in type 2 diabetes. *N Engl J Med*. 2008;358:2545-59.

ADVANCE Collaborative Group. Intensive blood glucose and vascular outcomes in patients with type 2 diabetes. *N Engl J Med*. 2008;358:2560-72.

American Association of Clinical Endocrinologists. *Endocr Pract.* 2007;13 (Suppl 1):1-68.

Bennett WL, Maruthur NM, Singh S, et al. Comparative effectiveness and safety of medications for type 2 diabetes: an update including new drugs and two-drug combination. *Ann Intern Med* 2011;154:602-13.

Chen JM, Rimm EB, Colditz GA, et al. Obesity, fat distribution, and weight gain as risk factors for clinical diabetes in men. *Diabetes Care* 1994;17:96-9.

Colditz GA, Willett WC, Rotnitzky A, et al. Weight gain as a risk factor for clinical diabetes in women. *Ann Intern Med.* 1995;22:481-6.

Currie CJ, Peters JP, Tynan A, et al. Survival as a function of HbA$_{1c}$ in people with type 2 diabetes: a retrospective cohort study. *Lancet.* 2010;375:481-9.

Dormandy JA, Charbonnel B, Eckland DJA, et al. Secondary prevention of macrovascular events in patients with type 2 diabetes in the PROactive study (PROspective pioglitAzone Clinical Trial in macroVascular Events): a randomised controlled trial. *Lancet.* 2005;366:1279-89.

Drucker DJ, Goldfine AB. Cardiovascular safety and diabetes drug development. *Lancet.* 2011:977-9.

Drucker DJ, Nauck MA. The incretin system: glucagon-like peptide-1 receptor agonists and dipeptidyl peptidase-4 inhibitors in type 2 diabetes. *Lancet.* 2006;368:1696-705.

Duckworth W, Abraira C, Moritz T, et al. Glucose control and vascular complications in veterans with type 2 diabetes. *N Engl J Med.* 2009;360:129-39.

Eckel RH, Grundy SM, Zimmet PZ. The metabolic syndrome. *Lancet.* 2005;365:1415-28.

European Diabetes Working Party for Older People 2001-2004. *Clinical guidelines for type 2 diabetes mellitus (older people). Available at:* http://eugms.org/index.php?pid=30. Accessed 2011 June 9

Gregg EW, Cheng YJ, Saydah S, et al. Trends in death rates among U.S. adults with and without diabetes between 1997 and 2006. *Diabetes Care* 2012;35:1252-57.

Holman RR, Paul SK, Bethel MA, et al. 10-Year follow-up of intensive glucose control in type 2 diabetes. *N Engl J Med.* 2008;359:1577-89.

Jarvis J, Skinner TC, Carey ME, Davies MJ. How can structured self-management patient education improve outcomes in people with type 2 diabetes? *Diabetes Obes Metab.* 2010;12:12-9.

Kahn SE, Haffner SM, Heise MA, et al. Glycemic durability of rosiglitazone, metformin or glyburide monotherapy. *N Engl J Med.* 2006;355:2427-43.

Kahn SE, Hull RL, Utzschneider KM. Mechanisms linking obesity to insulin resistance and type 2 diabetes. *Nature.* 2006;444:840-6.

Kelly TN, Bazzano LA, Fonseca VA, et al. Systematic review: glucose control and cardiovascular disease in type 2 diabetes. *Ann Intern Med.* 2009;151:394-403.

Mazzone T, Chait A, Plutzky J. Cardiovascular disease risk in type 2 diabetes mellitus: insights from mechanistic studies. *Lancet.* 2008;371:1800-9.

Nathan DM, Buse JB, Davidson MB, et al. Medical management of hyperglycaemia in type 2 diabetes mellitus: a consensus algorithm for the initiation and adjustment of therapy: a consensus statement from the American Diabetes Association and the European Association for the Study of Diabetes. *Diabetologia.* Epub 2008 Oct. 22. 2009;52:17-30.

Nissen SE, Wolski K. Effect of rosiglitazone on the risk of myocardial infarction and death from cardiovascular causes. *N Engl J Med.* 2007;356:2457-71.

Ray KK, Seshasai SR, Wijesuriya S, et al. Effect of intensive control of glucose on cardiovascular outcomes and death in patients with diabetes mellitus: a meta-analysis of randomised controlled trials. *Lancet.* 2009;373:1765-72.

Stumvoll M, Goldstein BJ, van Haeften TW. Type 2 diabetes: principles of pathogenesis and therapy. *Lancet.* 2005;365:1333-46.

Turnbull FM, Abraira C, Anderson RJ, et al. Intensive glucose control and macrovascular outcomes in type 2 diabetes. *Diabetologia.* 2009;52:2288-98.

UK Prospective Diabetes Study (UKPDS) Group. (UKPDS 16) Overview of six years' therapy of type 2 diabetes - a progressive disease UKPDS Group. *Diabetes.* 1995;44:1249-58.

UK Prospective Diabetes Study (UKPDS) Group. Intensive blood-glucose control with sulfonylureas or insulin compared with conventional treatment and risk of complications in patients with type 2 diabetes (UKPDS 33). *Lancet.* 1998a;352:837-53.

UK Prospective Diabetes Study (UKPDS) Group. Effect of intensive blood-glucose control with metformin on complications in overweight patients with type 2 diabetes (UKPDS 34). *Lancet.* 1998b;352:854-65.

Stratton IM, Adler AI, Neil HA, et al. Association of glycaemia with macrovascular and microvascular complications of Type 2 diabetes: prospective observational study. *BMJ.* 2000;321:405-12.

Wallace TM, Matthews DR. The drug treatment of type 2 diabetes. In: Pickup JC, Williams G, eds. Textbook of diabetes, 3rd edn. Oxford: Blackwell; 2003. pp. 45.1-18.

Zoungas S, de Galan BE, Ninomiya T, et al., ADVANCE Collaborative Group. Combined effects of routine blood pressure lowering and intensive glucose control on macrovascular and microvascular outcomes in patients with type 2 diabetes: new results from the ADVANCE trial. *Diabetes Care.* 2009;32:2068-74.

Chapter 2

Established classes of glucose-lowering drugs

1. Introduction

Newer drugs for the treatment of type 2 diabetes have to be positioned within an existing framework of more established therapies. There is half a century of clinical experience with biguanides and sulphonylureas. Drugs within these archetypal classes illustrate the potential for clinically important differences between individual compounds. These differences are reflected principally in safety and tolerability rather than appreciable differences in long-term efficacy, although there is some support for the latter.

The UK Prospective Diabetes Study (UKPDS) was completed just as a new class of oral glucose-lowering agents became available – the thiazolidinediones. The launch was inauspicious: severe hepatotoxicity ensured the rapid demise of the first member of the class to enter clinical practice – troglitazone. Issues of weight gain, oedema, risk of bone fractures and cardiac failure in susceptible patients apply to the remaining two drugs – rosiglitazone and pioglitazone. Moreover, new safety concerns have emerged in the past few years. Although they have become well established and widely used, the role of thiazolidinediones is being re-evaluated.

The progressive nature of type 2 diabetes was well demonstrated in the UKPDS. This translates into a need for combinations of glucose-lowering drugs in the majority of patients. In the UKPDS fewer than half of the participants treated with metformin or a sulphonylurea were at the target glycated haemoglobin (HbA_{1c}) level of 7.0% 3 years after diagnosis. Drugs from different classes tend to have additive rather than synergistic effects, and bringing blood glucose concentrations down into the physiological range remains difficult to achieve. All major classes of oral glucose-lowering agents, when used appropriately, reduce glycated haemoglobin concentrations by broadly similar degrees. Some data point to differences between classes but more robust long-term comparisons are required. These observations perhaps point to some fundamental deficits in our understanding of the heterogeneous mechanisms that lead to chronic hyperglycaemia. It is clear that genetic, epigenetic, behavioural and environmental factors conspire to produce a broad range of phenotypes. These factors account for some of the differences in individual responses to oral agents.

A. J. Krentz, *Drug Therapy for Type 2 Diabetes*,
DOI: 10.1007/978-1-908517-77-7_2,
© Springer International Publishing Switzerland 2012

2. Biguanides

Metformin (dimethylbiguanide) is the only biguanide available in most countries. Phenformin was tarnished by lactic acidosis and was withdrawn from the UK in the late 1970s. Metformin was introduced in the USA in 1995. While metformin carries a much lower risk of lactic acidosis than phenformin, clinicians are required to ensure that appropriate steps are taken to minimise the occurrence of this potentially life-threatening side-effect. Metformin is thought to be the most commonly prescribed oral glucose-lowering agent worldwide. The drug enjoyed a surge in use following the publication of the UKPDS; it is relatively inexpensive compared with newer drugs such as the thiazolidinediones and dipeptidyl peptidase 4 (DPP-4) inhibitors.

2.1 Mode of action

Metformin counters defective insulin action, i.e. it has insulin-sensitising properties but does not directly enhance insulin secretion. The drug exerts its effects on glucose metabolism by means of insulin-dependent and insulin-independent intracellular pathways, including the activation of adenosine 5′-monophosphate-activated protein kinase. Metformin appears to offer protection against the vascular complications of diabetes partly through mechanisms that are independent of its antihyperglycaemic properties (Box 2.1).

The full glucose-lowering efficacy of metformin requires the presence of insulin. The main effect is mediated by means of a reduction in hepatic glucose production (Figure 2.1). Metformin reduces gluconeogenesis by increasing hepatic insulin sensitivity, and by decreasing hepatic extraction of gluconeogenic substrates from the circulation; hepatic glycogenolysis is also decreased. To a lesser extent, metformin enhances insulin-stimulated glucose uptake in skeletal muscle cells where it promotes glycogen synthesis. Metformin directly suppresses fatty acid oxidation; this may be of benefit in patients with hypertriglyceridaemia. The actions of metformin on fatty acids permit increased utilisation of glucose as a cellular energy source.

2.2 Pharmacokinetics

Metformin is rapidly but incompletely absorbed from the gastrointestinal tract. The drug is not metabolised. There is little binding to plasma proteins. Compared with plasma, higher concentrations are achieved in cells of the gastrointestinal tract. The plasma half-life of metformin is approximately 6 h; urinary elimination is complete within approximately 12 h. Renal clearance occurs principally by tubular secretion. Cimetidine competes for renal clearance and can cause a clinically significant increase in plasma metformin concentrations.

Box 2.1: Metabolic and vascular effects of metformin

Antihyperglycaemic action
- *Suppresses hepatic glucose output*
- *Increases insulin-mediated glucose utilisation*
- *Decreases fatty acid oxidation*
- *Increases splanchnic glucose turnover*

Weight stabilisation or reduction

Improves lipid profile
- *Reduces hypertriglyceridaemia*
- *Lowers plasma fatty acids and LDL-cholesterol; raises HDL-cholesterol in some patients*

No risk of serious hypoglycaemia

Counters insulin resistance
- *Decreases endogenous or exogenous insulin requirements*
- *Reduces basal plasma insulin concentrations*

Vascular effects
- *Increased fibrinolysis*
- *Decreases plasminogen activator inhibitor 1 levels*
- *Improved endothelial function*

2.3 Indications and contraindications

Metformin does not cause weight gain and can aid efforts directed at weight loss; this makes it the preferred drug for overweight and obese patients. Metformin appears to have similar antihyperglycaemic efficacy in normal weight patients, although the evidence base is less robust. Because of the risk of drug accumulation the use of metformin in patients with marked impairment of renal function should be avoided. The threshold of glomerular filtration at which risk is deemed unacceptable continues to be debated; this exercise is fraught with uncertainties and the issue remains controversial. In the UK, it is recommended that the dose of metformin be reviewed if the estimated glomerular filtration rate (eGFR) falls below 45 ml/min and avoided if it is less than 30 ml/min. This caution reflects concerns about the most feared adverse event – lactic acidosis. The incidence is low, but mortality is high. The risk of lactic acidosis with metformin has long been the subject of debate. Some prescribers hold the view that the danger has been exaggerated. Further contraindications include significant cardiac or respiratory insufficiency, or any other condition predisposing to major tissue hypoxia, e.g. hypotension, major infection, acute myocardial infarction. Metformin should be avoided in patients with clinically significant liver disease or

Figure 2.1. Main sites of action of metformin contributing to glucose-lowering effect.

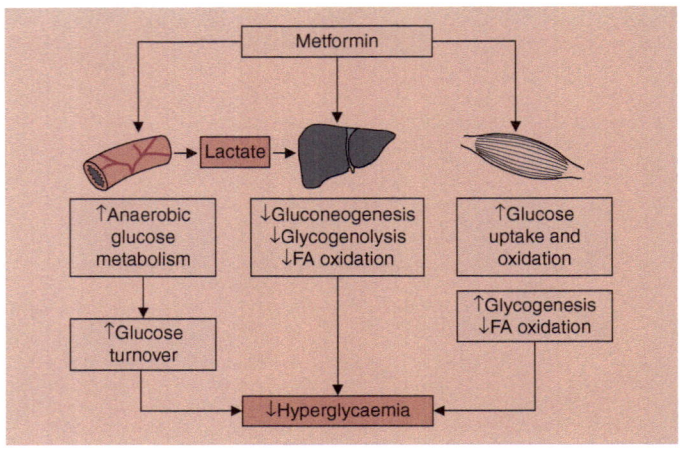

FA = Fatty acid.
Reproduced from Bailey and Krentz (2010), with permission.

alcohol dependency. Advanced age is not a contraindication to metformin in the absence of renal insufficiency and other exclusions. Ovulation can resume in women with polycystic ovary syndrome (PCOS). The use of metformin in PCOS is an unlicensed application in the absence of diabetes.

Unmodified tablet, liquid or powder formulations – so-called immediate release (IR) – should be taken during or immediately after meals in order to minimise gastrointestinal side-effects. Start with 500 or 850 mg once a day, or 500 mg twice a day divided between the morning and evening meals. Increase the dosage slowly – one tablet at a time – at approximately 1–2-week intervals. If glycaemic targets are not attained and an additional dose produces no further improvement, stepping down to the previous dose is sensible. The maximal effective dosage of metformin is approximately 2000 mg/day, although the maximum approved dose in some countries is higher.

Slow-release options (XR/SR/ER) are available in many countries. These can be taken once a day in the morning, or if necessary, morning and evening. Metformin is extensively used in combination with other classes of glucose-lowering agents, including insulin. Fixed-dose combination tablets are available in which metformin is combined with either a sulphonylurea (not available in the UK) or thiazolidinedione (pioglitazone in the UK) or certain DPP-4 inhibitors. Although metformin carries a negligible risk of hypoglycaemia as monotherapy or in combination with other low-risk drugs such as thiazolidinediones, it will potentiate the actions of insulin-releasing agents and insulin.

During the long-term use of metformin it is advised to check at least annually for the emergence of contraindications, particularly renal function. Metformin can reduce vitamin B_{12} absorption; this should be borne in mind during long-term therapy in individuals with other nutritional deficiencies. Metformin should be temporarily discontinued when intravenous radiographic contrast media are used because of the risk of an acute deterioration in renal function. Surgery with general anaesthesia carries risks of hypoxia and sepsis; substitution with insulin may be required as a safer option, with metformin being re-introduced when these risks have passed.

2.4 Efficacy

As monotherapy in patients not adequately controlled by lifestyle measures, optimally titrated metformin can be expected to reduce fasting plasma glucose by approximately 2–4 mmol/l; this corresponds to a decrease in HbA_{1c} of approximately 1–2%.

As discussed in Chapter 1, obese patients in the UKPDS who were commenced on metformin had a 39% reduced risk of myocardial infarction compared with conventional treatment (p = 0.01). Supporting the observations are studies demonstrating that metformin has beneficial effects on atherothrombotic risk markers (see Box 2.1). Recent results from the post-trial follow-up of UKPDS showed that the cardiovascular benefits of metformin were maintained (Table 2.1). However, a meta-analysis published in 2011 cast some doubt on specific beneficial effects of metformin on macrovascular events and mortality. There have been concerns that combination metformin plus sulphonylurea therapy might be associated with a higher risk of vascular complications than metformin monotherapy. A recent meta-analysis concluded that this combination significantly increased the risk of a cardiovascular event composite endpoint; however, there were no significant effects of this combination therapy on either cardiovascular mortality or all-cause mortality.

Although metformin is not indicated for the prevention of diabetes the US Diabetes Prevention Programme showed that metformin reduced the incidence of new cases of diabetes in overweight and obese subjects with impaired glucose tolerance by 33%, compared with a reduced risk of 58% using an intensive regimen of diet and exercise; the benefits were most evident in younger, more obese individuals.

2.5 Adverse effects

The main tolerability issue with metformin is abdominal discomfort and other gastrointestinal adverse effects, including diarrhoea. These are often transient side-effects that can be ameliorated by taking the drug with meals and

Table 2.1. **UKPDS 10-year follow-up study. Results for metformin compared with conventional treatment at end of UKPDS and after a median 8.5 years post-trial follow-up. Post-trial monitoring results showed continuing benefit of earlier metformin therapy, with maintenance of relative risk reductions – 'legacy effect'.**

Aggregate endpoint	1997	2007
Any diabetes-related endpoint		
Relative risk reduction	32%	21%
p value	0.0023	0.013
Myocardial infarction		
Relative risk reduction	39%	33%
p value	0.01	0.005
All-cause mortality		
Relative risk reduction	36%	27%
p value	0.011	0.002

UKPDS: UK Prospective Diabetes Study.
Reproduced from Holman et al. (2008) and Diabetes Trials Unit, University of Oxford, with permission.

titrating the dose slowly. Symptoms may remit if the dose is reduced, but approximately 10% of patients are unable to tolerate metformin at any dose. The most serious adverse event associated with metformin is lactic acidosis; as already mentioned this is rare, affecting approximately one in 100 000 patients, but its avoidance underpins the aforementioned contraindications to metformin, i.e. clinical situations that can lead to the accumulation of the drug, or produce major tissue hypoxia. Vitamin B_{12} deficiency is a potential hazard of long-term therapy that could impair peripheral nerve function. Periodic measurement of serum vitamin B_{12} status is recommended.

3. Sulphonylureas

Since their introduction in the 1950s, sulphonylureas have been used extensively for the treatment of type 2 diabetes. Modern examples include glibenclamide (known as glyburide in the USA and Canada), gliclazide, glipizide and glimepiride; these have largely replaced the first generation of sulphonylureas (Table 2.2). Sulphonylureas are relatively inexpensive. In the UK sulphonylureas and metformin are widely used but account for less than 50% of the total cost of glucose-lowering drugs.

3.1 Mode of action

Sulphonylureas stimulate insulin secretion from islet β cells (Figure 2.2). They bind to the cytosolic surface of the sulphonylurea receptor (SUR) 1, which forms part of a transmembrane complex with ATP-sensitive Kir6.2

potassium channels (K+ATP channels). This closes the K+ATP channel, reducing potassium efflux with membrane depolarisation resulting in calcium influx that in turn leads to the release of insulin from preformed granules. This generates the initial phase of insulin release which is followed by a more protracted second phase of insulin secretion. Because sulphonylureas will stimulate insulin release even when glucose concentrations are below normal they are capable of causing hypoglycaemia; fasting hypoglycaemia results mainly from the suppression of hepatic glucose production. Drugs with an intrinsically long duration of action, glibenclamide (glyburide) being the prime example, are associated with a higher risk of severe hypoglycaemia compared with shorter-acting sulphonylureas.

3.2 Pharmacokinetics

Sulphonylureas vary in their pharmacokinetic properties. They are all generally well absorbed, reaching peak plasma concentration in approximately 2–4 h. Sulphonylureas are generally highly bound to plasma proteins, which can lead to interactions with drugs such as salicylates, sulphonamides and warfarin. Displacement of protein-bound sulphonylureas can increase the risk of hypoglycaemia. Sulphonylureas are hepatically metabolised to active and inactive metabolites that are eliminated along with the parent drug in bile and urine. The formulation of some sulphonylureas has been altered to modify the duration of action. A micronised formulation of glibenclamide increases the rate of gastrointestinal absorption producing an earlier onset of action. A modified release formulation of gliclazide has been developed to allow once-daily dosing. This formulation is not available in all countries.

Table 2.2. Sulphonylureas.

Agent	Dose range (mg/day)	Duration of action (h)	Metabolites	Elimination
Tolbutamide	500–2000	6–10	Inactive	Urine 100%
Glipizide	5–20	6–16	Inactive	Urine ~70%
Gliclazide	40–320	12–20	Inactive	Urine ~65%
Gliclazide MR	30–120	18–24	Inactive	Urine ~65%
Glimepiride	1–6	12–>24	Active	Urine ~60%
Glibenclamide	2.5–15	12–>24	Active	Bile >50%
Chlorpropamide	100–500	24–50	Active	Urine >90%

New patients are not usually started on first-generation sulphonylureas (tolbutamide, chlorpropamide). Glibenclamide is also known as glyburide in the USA. Not all drugs or formulations listed are available in every country. Glimepiride is sometimes referred to as a third-generation sulphonylurea.
MR: Modified release.

Figure 2.2. Sulphonylureas act on the pancreatic β cells to stimulate insulin action. They bind to the cytosolic surface of the sulphonylurea receptor 1 (SUR-1), causing closure of ATP-sensitive Kir6.2 potassium channels, depolarising the plasma membrane, opening calcium channels and activating calcium-dependent signalling proteins that control insulin exocytosis.

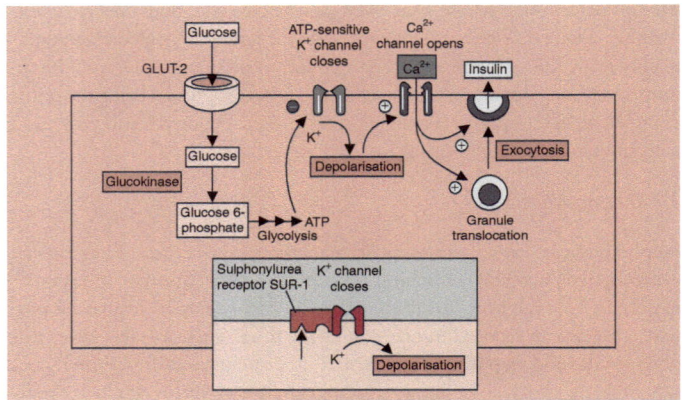

GLUT-2 = Glucose transporter 2.
Reproduced from Bailey and Krentz (2010), with permission.

3.3 Indications and contraindications

Sulphonylureas are widely used as monotherapy and in combination with metformin or a thiazolidinedione. They can also be used with an α-glucosidase inhibitor or a DPP-4 inhibitor. Combination therapy with insulin offers little advantage other than a somewhat lower insulin dosage. Combining a sulphonylurea with a different type of oral glucose-lowering agent generally brings an additive effect on glucose lowering, albeit with a higher risk of hypoglycaemia. Meglitinides, which like sulphonylureas act via the SUR-1 complex, generally offer no extra benefit beyond up-titration of the sulphonylurea.

Expert guidelines have tended to favour sulphonylureas as alternative first-line oral therapy when metformin is not appropriate or not tolerated. As sulphonylurea therapy is associated with weight gain, these agents have customarily been preferred for patients who are not overweight. Treatment should begin with a low dose. Up-titrate the dosage at 2–4-week intervals as required. The maximal blood glucose-lowering effect of an unmodified sulphonylurea is usually achieved at a dose well below the recommended maximum. Hypoglycaemia is the main limitation to dose escalation of sulphonylureas. Self-monitoring of blood glucose is recommended during the first few weeks of therapy. If evidence of hypoglycaemia occurs before the glycaemic target is achieved, or if a dosage increment produces no further glycaemic benefit, it is advisable to return to the previous dose. Additional or alternative therapy should be considered in these situations as appropriate.

3.4 Efficacy

As monotherapy in patients inadequately controlled by lifestyle measures, sulphonylureas can be expected to reduce fasting plasma glucose by approximately 2–4 mmol/l, equating to a decrease in HbA_{1c} of approximately 1–2%. The glucose-lowering effect of sulphonylureas is immediate, although efficacy is dependent on a sufficient reserve of β-cell function. A rapid deterioration of glycaemic control during sulphonylurea therapy occurs in approximately 5–10% of patients per annum. There is some evidence that there are differences between individual sulphonylureas in their capacity to maintain glycaemic control. As a class, the general trend is to a deterioration in control after an initial response, as demonstrated in the UKPDS. No drugs in the class have unequivocally been shown to reduce the progression to diabetes in patients with glucose intolerance. Sulphonylureas generally have little effect on blood lipids. Preliminary pharmacogenetic studies of genetic variants that influence enzymatic hepatic sulphonylurea metabolism and thus pharmacokinetics raise the possibility of identifying individuals more likely to respond well to sulphonylureas.

3.5 Adverse effects

Weight gain of approximately 1–4 kg, is common after the initiation of sulphonylurea therapy, with stabilisation by approximately 6 months. Sulphonylurea-induced weight gain is thought to be a consequence of the anabolic effects of increased plasma insulin concentrations. Hypoglycaemia is the most common and most serious adverse effect of sulphonylurea therapy. Although it is only rarely life threatening in patients with type 2 diabetes, with mild impairment of neural or motor functions. Patients treated with sulphonylureas, and their carers, should be given clear instructions on the prevention, recognition and management of hypoglycaemia. In the UKPDS approximately 20% of sulphonylurea-treated patients reported one or more episodes of symptomatic hypoglycaemia per annum; other studies suggest similar rates. Severe hypoglycaemia, i.e. requiring assistance from another person during sulphonylurea therapy, occurred in approximately 1% of patients annually in the UKPDS. Irregular meals, the concomitant use of other glucose-lowering drugs, excessive alcohol consumption, old age, unplanned or strenuous activity and drug interactions can increase the risk of hypoglycaemia. Patients who have already attained good glycaemic control are at greater risk. Chlorpropamide and glibenclamide (glyburide) are more likely to cause severe prolonged hypoglycaemia compared to newer drugs and their modified formulations. Severe sulphonylurea-induced hypoglycaemia requires prompt admission to hospital; there is an appreciable risk of fatality and a risk of residual neurological defects in survivors.

The suggestion from the UGDP (University Group Diabetes Program) study in the 1960s that tolbutamide might have a detrimental effect on cardiovascular outcomes remains unsubstantiated. Interest in the cardiovascular safety of sulphonylureas was re-ignited by the finding that two isoforms of the sulphonylurea receptor, SUR-2A and SUR-2B, are expressed in cardiac muscle and vascular smooth muscle, respectively. Whereas these isoforms lack the sulphonylurea binding site, they retain the benzamido binding site. Therefore, SUR-2A/B can only bind those sulphonylureas that contain a benzamido group, i.e. glibenclamide, glipizide and glimepiride. Sulphonylureas without a benzamido group, e.g. tolbutamide, chlorpropamide and gliclazide, show very little interaction with the cardiac and vascular SUR receptors. Theoretically, compounds with a benzamido group could interfere with ischaemic preconditioning and increase vascular contractility under unfavourable conditions, e.g. during myocardial ischaemia. However, there is no clear evidence that therapeutic concentrations of sulphonylureas exert such an effect. This controversy continues, and has been fuelled by reports from non-randomised studies suggesting that some, generally older, sulphonylureas are associated with a worse prognosis after myocardial infarction. Other data refute this assertion.

4. Meglitinides

Meglitinide, the non-sulphonylurea moiety of glibenclamide, which contains the benzamido group, stimulates insulin secretion. The pharmacokinetic properties of compounds developed from this observation provide a rapid and short duration release of insulin. Two agents, the meglitinide derivative repaglinide and the structurally related phenylalanine derivative nateglinide, have been available for a decade or so. Stimulation of first-phase insulin release during the prandial and early postprandial period helps control the rise in blood glucose after meals. The need for multiple daily dosages may detract from the flexibility of these agents, the latter being their main advantage over sulphonylureas. Prandial insulin releasers can be added to metformin or a thiazolidinedione. The meglitinides are relatively expensive compared with generic sulphonylureas.

4.1 Mode of action

Meglitinides bind to the SUR-1 benzamido site of the islet β cells. Whereas this site is distinct from the sulphonylurea site, the response is as for sulphonylureas, i.e. closure of the K^+ATP channel. It follows that there is generally no therapeutic advantage to combining these agonists. However, variations in binding affinities and duration of action between the classes may permit combination use of a meglitinide with a sulphonylurea to fit with an unusual meal pattern.

4.2 Pharmacokinetics

Repaglinide is rapidly absorbed with peak plasma concentration attained approximately 1 h after ingestion. Hepatic metabolism produces inactive metabolites, which are predominantly excreted in the bile (Table 2.3). If taken approximately 15 min before a meal, repaglinide produces a prompt insulin response that is complete by approximately 3 h. Nateglinide has a slightly faster onset and shorter duration of action.

4.3 Indications and contraindications

Repaglinide can be used as monotherapy in patients with inadequate glycaemic control after non-pharmacological measures; nateglinide is licensed for combination therapy with metformin in the UK. They can be useful for individuals with irregular lifestyles accompanied by unpredictable or missed meals. The lower risk of hypoglycaemia compared with sulphonylureas may be helpful in elderly patients. Repaglinide is best taken 15–30 min before a meal. Therapy should start with a low dose, e.g. 0.5 mg, unless the individual is transferring from another oral hypoglycaemic agent, in which case the dose should be 1 mg. Self-monitoring of postprandial blood glucose will guide up-titration every 2 weeks; the maximum dose is 4 mg before each main meal. When a meal is not consumed the corresponding dose of repaglinide is omitted. Repaglinide can be used, with caution, in patients with moderate degrees of renal impairment that preclude the use of sulphonylureas and metformin. Nateglinide has a faster onset and shorter duration of action than repaglinide. Caution is required in patients with hepatic disease.

4.4 Efficacy

Repaglinide and nateglinide produce dose-dependent increases in insulin concentrations and reduce postprandial hyperglycaemia. There is usually a

Table 2.3. The meglitinides: repaglinide and nateglinide.

Agent	Dose range (mg/meal)	Maximum daily dose (mg)	Duration of action (h)	Metabolites	Elimination
Repaglinide	0.5–4	16	4–6	Inactive	Bile ~90%
Nateglinide	60–180	540	3–5	One slightly active	Urine ~80%

lesser improvement in fasting hyperglycaemia. Reductions in HbA_{1c} are similar to or smaller than with sulphonylureas, as predicted by the shorter duration of action of the meglitinides. Added to metformin, they can reduce HbA_{1c} by an additional 0.5–1.5%. In the NAVIGATOR (Nateglinide and Valsartan in Impaired Glucose Tolerance Outcomes Research) trial, nateglinide up to 60 mg three times a day did not achieve a statistically significant reduction in new-onset diabetes in adults aged a mean of approximately 65 years with impaired glucose tolerance; a composite of cardiovascular events were not reduced by the drug.

4.5 Adverse effects

In general, hypoglycaemia is less frequent and less severe with meglitinides than with sulphonylureas. Plasma levels of repaglinide may be increased by gemfibrozil. Prandial insulin releasers cause an increase in body weight when used as initial monotherapy. In the NAVIGATOR trial body weight was approximately 0.4 kg greater in participants treated with nateglinide compared with placebo.

5. Thiazolidinediones

Thiazolidinediones are potent agonists of peroxisome proliferator-activated receptor gamma (PPARγ). The PPARγ-mediated transcriptional effects of thiazolidinediones on target genes improve whole-body insulin sensitivity. Troglitazone was the first thiazolidinedione to enter clinical use in 1997. However, the drug was associated with cases of fatal hepatotoxicity; it was withdrawn in 2000, having been available for only a few weeks in the UK. Two other thiazolidinediones, rosiglitazone and pioglitazone, which have not shown this hepatotoxicity, were introduced in the USA in 1999 and in Europe in 2000. Fixed-dose combinations of pioglitazone with metformin are available.

5.1 Mode of action

Most of the glucose-lowering efficacy of thiazolidinediones is thought to be achieved through increased insulin sensitivity in target tissues for insulin, primarily muscle, liver and adipose tissue. PPARγ is highly expressed in adipocytes, and to a lesser extent in muscle and liver. On activation PPARγ forms a heterodimeric complex with the retinoid X receptor and binds to a nucleotide sequence termed the peroxisome proliferator response element located in the promoter regions of PPAR-responsive genes. In conjunction with co-activators this alters the transcriptional activity of a range of genes, some of which are insulin sensitive, that participate in lipid and carbohydrate metabolism (Figure 2.3). Stimulation of PPARγ by thiazolidinediones promotes the differentiation of pre-adipocytes into mature adipocytes. These new small adipocytes are more sensitive to insulin, as demonstrated by the enhanced uptake of fatty acids and increased rates of lipogenesis. The reduced circulating level of fatty acids re-balances the glucose–fatty acid–Randle cycle, facilitating glucose utilisation in muscle. In the liver, reduced fatty acid availability serves to decrease excessive rates of hepatic gluconeogenesis. Ectopic lipid deposition in muscle and liver is reduced, whereas glucose uptake into adipose tissue and skeletal muscle is increased, by means of cellular insulin-sensitive glucose transporters. The putative contribution to improved insulin sensitivity resulting from the reduced production of adipocyte-derived pro-inflammatory cytokines is less well established. Thiazolidinediones increase the production of adiponectin, an adipocytokine that enhances insulin action and exerts potentially beneficial effects directly on the vasculature.

Thiazolidinediones, like metformin, can be classed as antihyperglycaemic agents – they do not usually cause hypoglycaemia as monotherapy. They require the presence of sufficient insulin to generate a maximal blood glucose-lowering effect. A predictable effect of improved insulin sensitivity is that plasma insulin concentrations are lowered by thiazolidinediones. The secretion of proinsulin and other less potent insulin precursors is reduced. Animal

Figure 2.3. Mechanism of action of a thiazolidinedione on an adipocyte.

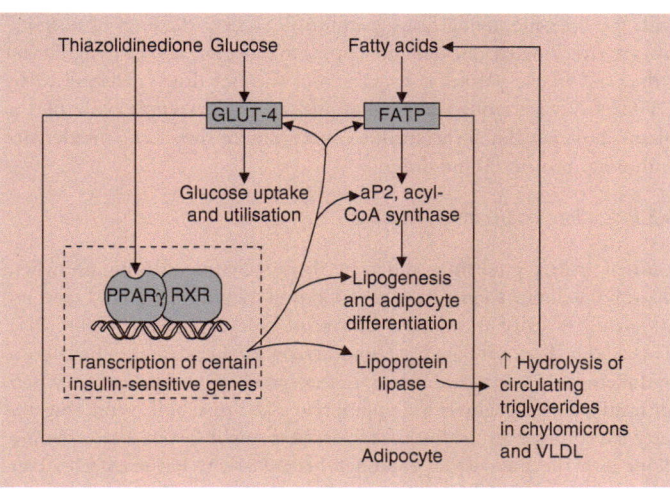

aP2 = Adipocyte fatty acid binding protein; CoA = coenzyme A; FATP = fatty acid transporter protein; GLUT-4 = glucose transporter 4; PPARγ = peroxisome proliferator-activated receptor gamma; RXR = retinoid X receptor; VLDL = very low-density lipoprotein; ↑ indicates increase.

Reproduced from Krentz and Bailey (2005), with permission.

Table 2.4. The thiazolidinediones: pioglitazone and rosiglitazone.

Agent	Dose range (mg/day)	Duration of action (h)	Metabolites	Elimination
Pioglitazone	15–45	~24	Active	Bile >60%
Rosiglitazone	4–8	~24	Inactive	Urine ~64%

studies generated hope that the long-term viability of islet β cells might be stabilised or improved. While no firm evidence for such an effect in humans has been found, the glucose-lowering effect of thiazolidinediones has been somewhat more durable than comparator drugs in some studies.

5.2 Pharmacokinetics

The gastrointestinal absorption of rosiglitazone and pioglitazone is rapid and near complete. Peak concentrations are attained at approximately 1–2 h. Both drugs are extensively metabolised by the liver (Table 2.4). Rosiglitazone is metabolised mainly by cytochrome P450 isoform CYP2C8 to metabolites with a plasma half-life of approximately 100–160 h; these are regarded as having no or minor activity and are eliminated in the urine. Pioglitazone is metabolised predominantly by CYP2C8 and CYP3A4 to active metabolites that are eliminated in the bile. Rosiglitazone interacts with the lipid-modifying drug gemfibrozil, causing the level of rosiglitazone to rise. Pioglitazone does not appear to cause any clinically significant reductions in the plasma concentrations of other drugs metabolised by CYP3A4. Rosiglitazone and pioglitazone are almost completely bound to plasma proteins, but at therapeutic concentrations there is no interference with other protein-bound drugs.

5.3 Indications and contraindications

Current expert guidelines differ in their recommendations on where thiazolidinediones should be placed. Clinical trials have explored their use at several stages of the natural history of type 2 diabetes (Figure 2.4). Thiazolidinediones are used as monotherapy, either as drugs of first choice or if metformin is inappropriate or not tolerated, and for patients in whom an insulin secretagogue is less appropriate. The metabolic syndrome and fatty liver disease are additional factors that might favour a thiazolidinedione over the alternatives. Although hepatotoxicity has not been a concern with either rosiglitazone or pioglitazone, the troglitazone experience prompted vigilance concerning liver function by measuring serum alanine aminotransferase before starting therapy and periodically thereafter. Pre-existing liver disease, the development of clinical hepatic dysfunction or elevated alanine aminotransferase levels more than 2.5 times the upper limit of the normal range are contraindications to thiazolidinediones. It may seem somewhat counterintuitive that recent studies have suggested that this class of drug might be useful for the treatment of non-alcoholic steatohepatitis; more data are required.

Thiazolidinediones require several weeks to exert a maximal effect on glucose levels. They are often used in combination with other glucose-lowering drugs, particularly metformin. As a result of their slow onset of action, substituting thiazolidinedione for either a sulphonylurea or metformin can result in a temporary deterioration in glycaemic control. Combining pioglitazone with insulin can improve glycaemic control while reducing insulin dosages, especially in obese patients. This approach should, however, be approached with caution: peripheral oedema is more common and concerns about precipitating heart failure are heightened. The propensity of thiazolidinediones to cause fluid retention and to expand plasma volume is a major safety issue. This is associated with minor reductions in blood haemoglobin concentrations. The use of thiazolidinediones is thus contraindicated in patients with heart failure. The precise exclusion

Figure 2.4. Overview of recent studies of thiazolidinediones and the natural history of the development and progression of type 2 diabetes.

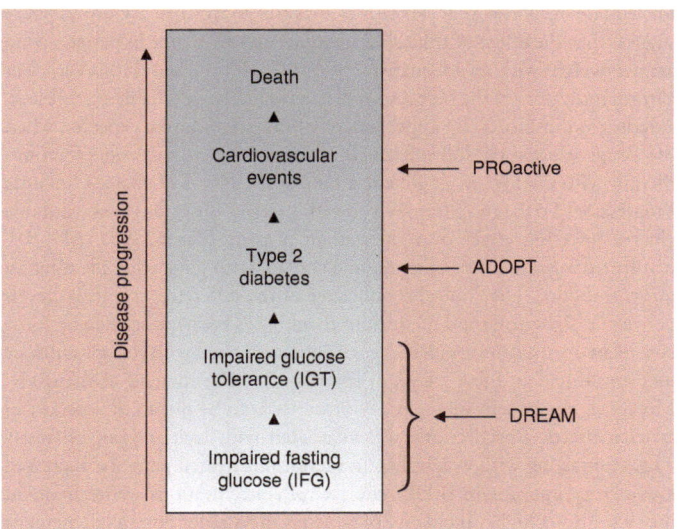

ADOPT = A Diabetes Outcome Progression Trial; DREAM = Diabetes Reduction Assessment with Ramipril and Rosiglitazone Medication; PROactive = PROspective pioglitAzone Clinical Trial In macro-Vascular Events.
Redrawn with permission from Krentz (2009).

criteria, based on cardiac status, vary in detail between countries. Appropriate clinical monitoring is important, especially for patients considered at higher risk of cardiac failure and those showing marked initial weight gain.

Hopes were raised that improved insulin sensitivity and positive effects on vascular risk markers would translate into cardioprotection. However, in 2007 a major controversy about the cardiovascular safety of rosiglitazone ignited. A meta-analysis of several clinical trials suggested that rosiglitazone increased the risk of myocardial infarction during the first 6–12 months of therapy. As discussed below, continuing doubts about this issue eventually led to withdrawal of rosiglitazone in Europe and instigation of tight restrictions on use of the drug in the USA.

Providing there are no contraindications, thiazolidinediones can be used in the elderly. They can also be considered for patients with mild renal impairment, while appreciating the potential for oedema given the possibility of fluid retention. In women with anovulatory PCOS, thiazolidinedione therapy can cause ovulation to resume; this risk should be explained to the patient. Thiazolidinediones should not be continued during pregnancy.

5.4 Efficacy

Thiazolidinediones produce a slowly generated glucose-lowering effect. An inadequate response may take 2–3 months to confirm. Clinical trials suggest that the effect of thiazolidinediones may be better in patients who are overweight with an adequate reserve of β-cell function. However, clear clinical indicators of the best responders have not been reliably established. A reduction in HbA_{1c} by approximately 0.5–1.5% can be expected when the drugs exert their full effects. In a long-term comparison of monotherapy with metformin or glibenclamide (ADOPT; A Diabetes Outcome Progression Trial), rosiglitazone showed a slower onset but more durable glucose-lowering effect over more than 3 years (Figure 2.5). ADOPT confirmed a gradual loss of glycaemic control with glibenclamide after an initial response. The clinical significance of the difference in HbA_{1c} levels between rosiglitazone and metformin therapy has been questioned by some commentators; a similar percentage of patients treated with rosliglitazone or metformin had an HbA_{1c} level of less than 7.0% at the end of the study. Moreover, the benefit in glucose control needs to be put in the context of adverse effects. Rosiglitazone was associated with weight gain, of nearly 5 kg, contrasting with weight loss in metformin-treated patients. Increased low-density lipoprotein (LDL) cholesterol concentrations, more frequent use of statins, a higher incidence of oedema and a reduction in haematocrit were observed with rosiglitazone. Some evidence of a more sustained glycaemic response, cf. sulphonylureas, has also been shown for pioglitazone.

Thiazolidinediones reduce circulating non-esterified fatty acid concentrations. The effects on other components of the plasma lipid profile

Figure 2.5. Fasting plasma glucose (A) and glycated haemoglobin (B) over time from ADOPT (A Diabetes Outcome Progression Trial).

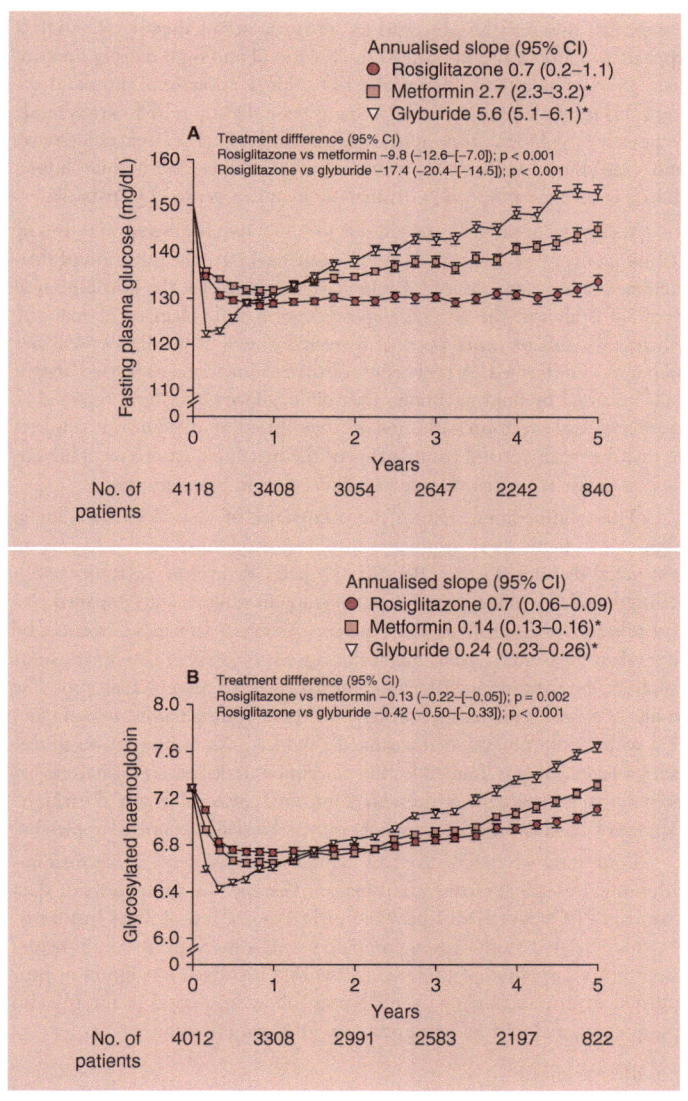

*Significant difference between rosiglitazone and other treatment groups.

Reproduced from Kahn et al. (2006), with permission.

are variable; this has fed into the recent controversy about the cardiovascular safety profiles of rosiglitazone and pioglitazone. Rosiglitazone tends to cause a small rise in total cholesterol concentration, stabilising by approximately 3 months; this may be obscured by adequate statin therapy. The effect appears to reflect a rise in both LDL-cholesterol and high-density lipoprotein (HDL) cholesterol, leaving the LDL : HDL-cholesterol ratio and the total : HDL-cholesterol ratio little changed or slightly raised. Triglyceride responses vary. Pioglitazone appears to have little effect on total cholesterol, and consistently reduced triglyceride concentrations. Both thiazolidinediones reduce the proportion of small dense atherogenic LDL particles.

Weight gain, similar in magnitude to sulphonylurea therapy, i.e. 1–4 kg stabilising over 6–12 months, is usually observed after the initiation of thiazolidinedione therapy. Several studies have indicated that the distribution of body fat is altered: the visceral adipose depot is little changed or reduced, whereas the subcutaneous depot is increased as new small, insulin-sensitive adipocytes are formed. A proportion of thiazolidinedione-associated weight gain is caused by fluid retention. Thiazolidinediones have been reported to exert beneficial effects on a selection of atherothrombotic risk markers, indices of vascular reactivity and components of the metabolic syndrome. Thiazolidinedione use is associated with a small decrease in blood pressure.

Thiazolidinediones reduce the occurrence of new-onset diabetes in high-risk individuals with glucose intolerance or those with a history of gestational diabetes. In the DREAM (Diabetes Reduction Assessment with Ramipril and Rosiglitazone Medication) study in subjects with impaired glucose tolerance or fasting hyperglycaemia progression to diabetes was reduced by more than 50% after 3 years, but at the expense of a higher rate of new heart failure in the rosiglitazone (0.5%) compared with placebo (0.1%) arm. The results of a small study using relatively low doses of rosiglitazone in combination with metformin also demonstrated a reduced risk of progression to diabetes. Neither drug is licensed for the prevention of diabetes. Pioglitazone has been shown to reduce the progression of impaired glucose tolerance albeit at the expense of a higher incidence of weight gain and oedema compared to placebo.

Long-term glycaemic control can be achieved with a metformin–sulphonylurea–pioglitazone combination therapy. In an analysis of data from the PROactive (PROspective pioglitAzone Clinical Trial In macro-Vascular Events) study, when compared with a metformin–sulphonylurea–placebo combination there was a twofold increased likelihood of progression to insulin therapy over a 3-year follow-up period in the placebo group compared with pioglitazone using this combination.

5.5 Adverse effects

Recent safety concerns have centred on cardiovascular safety and bone metabolism. The favourable impact of thiazolidinediones on cardiovascular risk factors raised hopes of reducing the risk of atherothrombotic events. In PROactive the primary composite endpoint was not significantly reduced, whereas a prespecified composite secondary cardiovascular endpoint (all-cause mortality, non-fatal myocardial infarction and stroke) indicated benefits in high-risk patients with pre-existing cardiovascular disease (Figure 2.6). In the PERISCOPE (Pioglitazone Effect on Regression of Intravascular Sonographic Coronary Obstruction Prospective Evaluation) study, a decrease in atheroma volume was observed in pioglitazone-treated subjects compared with an increase in glimepiride-treated patients using coronary intravascular ultrasound. More patients taking glimepiride developed hypoglycaemia and angina, whereas pioglitazone-treated patients were more likely to develop oedema and gain bodyweight, or sustain skeletal fractures. The evidence for pioglitazone thus suggests vasculoprotective effects, albeit at the cost of an increased incidence of well recognised side-effects.

The European Medicines Agency (EMA) approved the use of pioglitazone and rosiglitazone in 2000, but required post-marketing cardiovascular outcome studies because of concerns over the increased risk of heart failure and other cardiovascular effects. In 2007, publication of the aforementioned meta-analysis of clinical trial data suggested a significant 43% increase in the risk of myocardial infarction (p = 0.03) along with a non-significant 64% rise in cardiovascular death among patients taking rosiglitazone. Additional meta-analyses proved inconclusive. A warning was added to the US labelling for rosiglitazone in 2007. This stated that the drug was associated with an increased risk of myocardial ischaemic events, such as angina or myocardial infarction, in some patients. It was recommended that the drug be avoided in patients treated with insulin (reflecting a higher risk of myocardial ischaemia in trials in which rosiglitazone was added to insulin) or nitrates. The results of the RECORD (Rosiglitazone Evaluated for Cardiovascular Outcomes) study were more reassuring with respect to cardiovascular safety. The issue of the cardiovascular safety of rosiglitazone had assumed a highly charged political dimension by this point. Pressure was mounting on regulatory authorities that was to lead to decisive action in 2010. Critics pointed to methodological shortcomings in RECORD. This was a non-inferiority trial of over 4000 patients who have inadequate glycaemic control while receiving either metformin or a sulphonylurea. Patients were assigned to add-on rosiglitazone to a combination of metformin plus a sulphonylurea. The primary outcome, cardiovascular hospitalisation or cardiovascular death, was similar between the groups. More patients in the rosiglitazone group required additional therapies to maintain glycaemic control. Skeletal fractures and heart failure were seen more often with rosiglitazone. The ADOPT study also reported an increase in upper limb fractures in women treated with rosiglitazone. Lower limb fractures were increased in the foot but there was no difference in the number of hip fractures. A review of the safety database for pioglitazone has revealed a similar increase in distal bone

Figure 2.6. Kaplan–Meier curve of time to progression to: **(A)** primary composite endpoint (death from any cause, non-fatal myocardial infarction, including silent myocardial infarction, stroke, acute coronary syndrome, leg amputation, coronary revascularisation, or revascularisation of the leg); and **(B)** main secondary endpoint (death from any cause, non-fatal myocardial infarction, excluding silent myocardial infarction, or stroke), from **PRO**active (**PRO**spective piogl**it**Azone **C**linical **T**rial **I**n macro**V**ascular **E**vents).

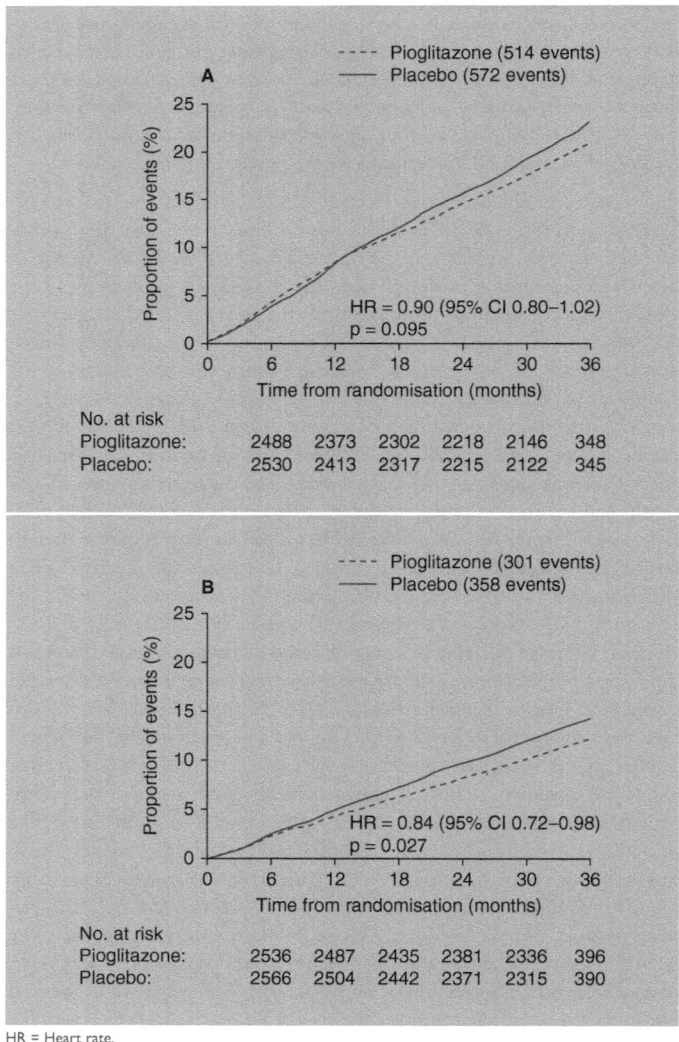

HR = Heart rate.

Reproduced from Dormandy et al. (2005), with permission.

fractures in women. Current data suggest that thiazolidinediones may cause bone loss, the effect being most prominent in postmenopausal women. Clinicians must therefore consider the risk of fractures among candidates for thiazolidinedione therapy. Postulated mechanisms leading to bone fragility include the inhibition of osteoblast activity and local adipogenesis. Caution should be exercised in patients considered to be predisposed to osteopenia.

The aforementioned issue of the cardiovascular safety concerns with rosiglitazone reached its conclusion in September 2010. Following the publication of additional studies that lent further support to these concerns the EMA recommended suspension of rosiglitazone. The US Food and Drug Administration (FDA) instituted a strict policy designed to restrict use of the drug but did not demand its withdrawal. These decisions were made in recognition of the availability of pioglitazone as an alternative not tarnished by questions of myocardial safety.

The BARI 2D (Bypass Angioplasty Revascularisation Investigation in Type 2 Diabetes) study included patients with type 2 diabetes and stable ischaemic heart disease. Randomisation was to early coronary revascularisation plus intensive medical therapy or intensive medical therapy alone. In a second randomisation strategy, patients were assigned to either insulin-provision therapy – an insulin secretagogue or insulin – or rosiglitazone. Survival rates were similar between the groups, and the results have been interpreted as reassuring with respect to the safety of rosiglitazone in high-risk cardiac patients. A recently published observational study using data from UK general practice concluded that pioglitazone was superior to rosiglitazone in mortality outcomes. Methodological limitations demand a cautious interpretation of these data. Since mid-2007, prescriptions for rosiglitazone in England have declined; by late 2008 pioglitazone was the most commonly prescribed thiazolidinedione.

In 2011 regulators responded to reports of a small increase in bladder cancer with pioglitazone. The FDA and EMA added warnings to the label with the aim of reducing exposure of high-risk patients to the drug. An association between macular oedema and glitazones has been reported. Familial polyposis coli is a theoretical contraindication to glitazone therapy.

6. Alpha-glucosidase inhibitors

Acarbose was introduced into clinical practice in the early 1990s. Two other agents, miglitol and voglibose, are available in some countries.

6.1 Mode of action

Alpha-glucosidase inhibitors competitively inhibit the activity of α-glucosidase enzymes in the brush border of the enterocytes lining the intestinal villi (Figure 2.7). They bind to the enzymes with high affinity preventing the cleavage of disaccharides and oligosaccharides to monosaccharides. In patients whose diet includes complex carbohydrates, α-glucosidase inhibitors can reduce postprandial glucose concentrations by retarding the absorption of monosaccharides. Each α-glucosidase inhibitor exhibits somewhat different affinities for the range of α-glucosidase enzymes. By transferring glucose absorption more distally α-glucosidase inhibitors may alter the release of glucose-dependent incretin hormones that enhance nutrient-induced insulin secretion. In practice, α-glucosidase inhibitors reduce postprandial insulin concentrations; this is considered to be secondary to lowering postprandial blood glucose levels.

6.2 Pharmacokinetics

Amylases and intestinal bacteria degrade acarbose. Less than 2% of the drug is absorbed together with some intestinal degradation products. Eliminatation occurs within 24 h, mainly in urine. Miglitol is almost completely absorbed and eliminated unchanged in the urine.

6.3 Indications and contraindications

Alpha-glucosidase inhibitors can be used as monotherapy, being preferred for patients with predominantly postprandial hyperglycaemia. More

Figure 2.7. Mode of action of α-glucosidase inhibitors. Alpha-glucosidase inhibitors competitively inhibit the activity of α-glucosidase enzymes in the brush border of enterocytes lining the intestinal villi, preventing these enzymes from cleaving disaccharides and oligosaccharides into monosaccharides. This delays carbohydrate digestion.

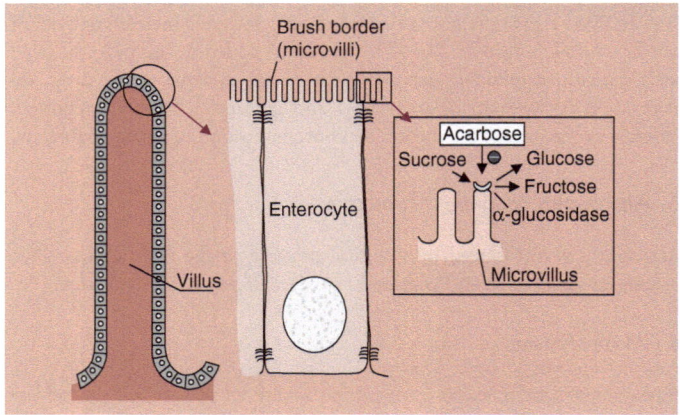

Redrawn from Bailey and Krentz (2010), with permission.

commonly, α-glucosidase inhibitors are added to other therapies when postprandial hyperglycaemia persists. Acarbose can prevent, or delay, the progression of impaired glucose tolerance to type 2 diabetes in high-risk patients; this is not a licensed indication. Voglibose, in addition to lifestyle modification, reduced the development of type 2 diabetes in a clinical trial of Japanese individuals with impaired glucose tolerance. Alpha-glucosidase inhibitors are contraindicated in patients with a history of chronic intestinal disease. High dosages of acarbose, i.e. 200 mg three times a day, may reversibly increase liver enzyme concentrations.

6.4 Initiation and dose titration

Alpha-glucosidase inhibitors should be taken with meals, starting with a low dose, e.g. 50 mg daily of acarbose, up-titrated over several weeks. Hypoglycaemia is unlikely when α-glucosidase inhibitors are used as monotherapy. Gastrointestinal symptoms, which demand slow dose titration, tend to subside with time. Nonetheless, in practice tolerability is frequently a major issue in UK practice. In contrast, acarbose is more widely used in some other countries; China for example.

6.5 Efficacy

As monotherapy, these agents can reduce peak postprandial glucose concentrations by 1–4 mmol/l. The effects on fasting hyperglycaemia are less impressive, usually less than 1 mmol/l. The decrease in glycated haemoglobin is approximately 0.5–1.0%, if a relatively high dose is tolerated. The theoretical cardiovascular benefits of preferentially reducing postprandial hyperglycaemia found support in the STOP–NIDDM (Study to Prevent Non-Insulin-Dependent Diabetes Mellitus) trial; these observations await confirmation.

6.6 Adverse effects

Alpha-glucosidase inhibitors do not cause weight gain or hypoglycaemia and may lower plasma triglycerides. Combining an α-glucosidase inhibitor with a sulphonylurea may, however, increase the risk of hypoglycaemia compared with sulphonylurea monotherapy. Oral treatment for hypoglycaemia under these circumstances should rely on glucose, not sucrose. In the STOP–NIDDM trial approximately 30% of acarbose-treated patients compared with approximately 20% on placebo discontinued treatment prematurely. If the dosage is too high relative to the amount of complex carbohydrate ingested, oligosaccharides pass undigested into the large bowel. When fermented, flatulence, abdominal discomfort, and sometimes diarrhoea ensue.

7. Fixed dose combinations of orally active drugs

The use of fixed dose combinations of oral glucose-lowering agents with different mechanisms of action has become widely accepted. These are designed to provide bioequivalence and thereby similar efficacy; minor adjustments to the formulation may enable some extra blood glucose-lowering efficacy. Fixed-dose combinations can offer convenience, reduce the treatment burden and simplify daily medication regimens. These may increase patient adherence – a major problem with a long-term condition such as type 2 diabetes, which brings little in the way of symptoms unless hyperglycaemia is marked. Lower doses of two different types of agents rather than a high dose of one agent may provide efficacy while reducing dose-related side effects. Fixed-dose combinations of metformin with several other classes are available. Although single tablets could reduce titration flexibility, most of the commonly used dosage combinations are available. Any combination therapy necessitates the same cautions and contraindications that apply to each active component.

8. Principles of insulin therapy in type 2 diabetes

Clinical experience with insulin is unrivalled among glucose-lowering drug therapies. Clinical trials have demonstrated delayed onset and progression of vascular complications with reduced morbidity and mortality in patients with type 2 diabetes. Many uncertainties about the optimal use of insulin, however, surround its use in clinical practice. Advantages and disadvantages are presented in Box 2.2. In recent decades, developments in insulin manufacture have led to successive refinements, initially with improvements in purity, and then with the mass production of human sequence insulin. These advances have been coupled with advances in injection devices, making the practicalities of self-administration less daunting. However, subcutaneous insulin injection can only partially mimic the exquisitely sensitive response of normal β cells to glucose and other endogenous regulators. Thus fundamental problems with insulin replacement therapy remain unresolved (Box 2.3).

Recent innovations have provided new therapeutic options for type 2 diabetes. Current data and clinical experience indicate that some of these new therapies can replace or delay the need for insulin treatment. The inexorable decline in β-cell function in type 2 diabetes ultimately renders oral agents ineffective. Insulin restores circulating levels of the hormone regardless of the endogenous production or duration of diabetes. Insulin has beneficial effects on insulin sensitivity, vascular function, dyslipidaemia and biomarkers that presage vascular damage. The glucose-lowering effects of insulin are unmatched; no maximum dose exists. Even patients with major metabolic disturbances respond to adequate doses, although in practice arbitrary limits are usually reached. Insulin can be combined with

Box 2.2: Insulin therapy in type 2 diabetes

Advantages

- *Unrivalled glucose lowering*
- *Flexibility in dosage and timing*
- *Rapidly adaptable regimens to suit changing clinical circumstances*
- *Evidence base of microvascular and macrovascular complication reduction*
- *Well-documented tolerability and safety profile*
- *Can be combined with many other glucose-lowering therapies*
- *Strategies to reduce weight gain and the risk of hypoglycaemia have been developed*

Disadvantages

- *Requires injection in standard formulation*
- *Frequent self-monitoring of blood glucose is necessary*
- *Risk of severe hypoglycaemia increases with duration of insulin therapy*
- *Day to day adjustments requires a high level of engagement by the patient*
- *Adequate knowledge about insulin use and safety issues is required*
- *Weight gain is common when insulin is initiated*
- *High doses may be necessary in patients with more severe degrees of insulin resistance*

a range of blood glucose-lowering agents. Insulin analogues (rapid-acting lispro and aspart, long-acting detemir and prolonged duration insulin glargine) are genetically engineered novel molecules. They offer some advantages over human insulin with improved pharmacokinetics (Table 2.5 and Figure 2.8). In practice, however, neither insulin glargine nor insulin detemir always give full 24-h coverage. These analogues approximate the stable, basal, secretion of insulin that normally accounts for approximately 50% of daily production. Insulin analogues can be formulated to provide biphasic pre-mixed options suitable for two or more daily injections. Insulin analogues are more expensive than human sequence insulins.

8.1 Basal insulin analogues

Insulin glargine has additional arginine molecules (B31 arginine and B32 arginine) located at the C-terminus of the B-chain, that confer additional positive charges thereby altering the isoelectric point. In addition, asparagine is replaced by arginine at A21 to confer stability. Glargine was designed to avoid the peak insulin concentration typically observed with conventional longer-acting insulins such as lente. Insulin glargine shows the following action profile: onset at approximately 90 min; prolonged plateau, rather than the peak of action with isophane insulin; duration of approximately 24 h, or longer.

Whereas insulin glargine is soluble at acid pH in the vial, when injected subcutaneously it forms a microprecipitate at the injection site

Box 2.3: Limitations inherent to insulin therapy

- *After subcutaneous injection, absorption delivers insulin into the systemic rather than portal circulation. This results in equivalent plasma insulin concentrations in both compartments; normal physiology maintains a gradient in which portal levels are much higher as a result of first-pass hepatic extraction.*

- *Suboptimal matching of delivery peak and decline of insulin concentrations compared with endogenous secretion results in suboptimal glucose profiles with the risk of hypoglycaemia as a result of continuing insulin action that is inappropriate to plasma glucose.*

- *It is not possible to mimic the endogenous surge of insulin into the portal circulation at the beginning of a meal; this first phase of insulin secretion promptly suppresses hepatic glucose production.*

- *Plasma insulin levels cannot be altered in response to fasting or exercise once an injection has been given; extra carbohydrate may be required.*

- *Controlling fasting plasma glucose concentrations by suppressing hepatic glucose production is difficult without inducing hypoglycaemia during the night. Prolonged duration insulin analogues offer an advantage over isophane insulin as they largely avoid the peak of insulin action that can lead to nocturnal hypoglycaemia. The latter is not always clinically apparent.*

- *Day-to-day variability in the absorption of intermediate duration insulin may be problematical in individual patients. This is reduced with prolonged duration insulin analogues permitting more predictable responses for a given daily dose.*

(because the latter is at a slightly alkaline, physiological pH). The stability of this microprecipitate slows the absorption of insulin into the circulation, which means that a single daily injection can provide a fairly stable level of insulin over a 24-h period, more closely mimicking the basal component of insulin secretion in healthy individuals. Glargine is rapidly converted to metabolites, predominantly M1 (~90-95%), with similar potency. 'Basal' insulin secretion accounts for approximately half of all daily insulin secretion, the rest being secreted in response to meals. The peakless action of glargine has been associated with a reduced incidence of hypoglycaemia, especially nocturnal episodes.

Insulin determir was introduced in the UK in 2004. This analogue has a C14 fatty acyl group attached to the B-chain (B29 lysine) of the insulin molecule, which binds to albumin, while the B30 threonine has been deleted. Detemir has a more evident peak of action, but it has been reported to produce predictable effects on glycaemic control, with little day-to-day variability. This may be an advantage in some patients when the attainment of glycaemic targets are proving difficult. The duration of action is up to 24 h depending on the dose, with higher doses tending to prolong the duration of action. There are reports of fewer episodes of hypoglycaemia and less weight gain with detemir compared with other insulins. Higher doses of detemir may be required to achieve equivalent glucose lowering, even though a unit of detemir contains four times as much insulin as other insulins. In some patients insulin detemir causes less local discomfort at injection sites.

The rationale for insulin, and practical steps for its initiation and intensification are discussed in the National Institute for Health and Clinical Excellence (NICE) clinical guideline 87; this guideline also considers the role of insulin glargine and insulin detemir (see Chapter 4). There has been a move away from starting therapy with isophane (neutral protamine Hagedorn; NPH) insulin, as currently advocated by NICE, in favour of insulin glargine and insulin detemir. Clinical trial data suggests benefits of insulin analogues over NPH insulin with respect to frequency of nocturnal hypoglycaemia. The 2009 American Association of Clinical Endocrinologists/American College of Endocrinology consensus panel comes down firmly against NPH insulin citing an inferior pharmacokinetic profile and excessive intra-individual day-to-day variability. Many options for the initiation, optimisation and intensification of insulin therapy have been published; the plurality of approaches reflects the choice of pharmacokinetic options. Insulin regimens are selected and adjusted on a case-by-case basis. Compared with older insulins, modern approaches to insulin therapy can help achieve metabolic targets with lower risks of the well-known adverse effects of therapy,

Table 2.5. Timing of metabolic effects for a selection of insulin preparations.

Insulin	Time of glucose-lowering effect (hours)		
	Onset	Peak	Duration
Rapid acting			
Insulin lispro	0–0.15	0.5–1.5	3–5
Insulin aspart	0–0.15	0.5–1.5	3–5
Insulin glulisine	0–0.15	0.5–1.5	3–5
Short acting			
Human soluble	0.25–1	1.5–4	5–9
Intermediate			
NPH (isophane)	0.5–2	3–6	8–14
Prolonged duration			
Insulin glargine	1–6	—	12–26
Insulin detemir	1–4	6–18	8–24

NPH: Neutral protamine Hagedorn.
Times are approximate and may vary between individuals, within individuals from day to day, and with dosage. Higher doses may prolong duration of action. Insulin degludec, a novel ultra-long acting analogue approved in some countries in 2102, has a duration of action of approximately 40 hours. Flexibility of daily dosing time and lower day-to-day variability are reported potential advantages. Ultra-long analogues may permit less than daily dosing.

Figure 2.8. Commonly used insulins in the UK. Action profiles are approximate and may differ between and within individual patients. Intra-individual day-to-day variation can be problematical with isophane (NPH) insulins. Insulin glargine, and in particular insulin detemir, show more predictable plasma levels as a result of less variable absorption. These analogues largely avoid the peak of insulin action observed with isophane insulin permitting the up-titration of doses with less risk of hypoglycaemia.

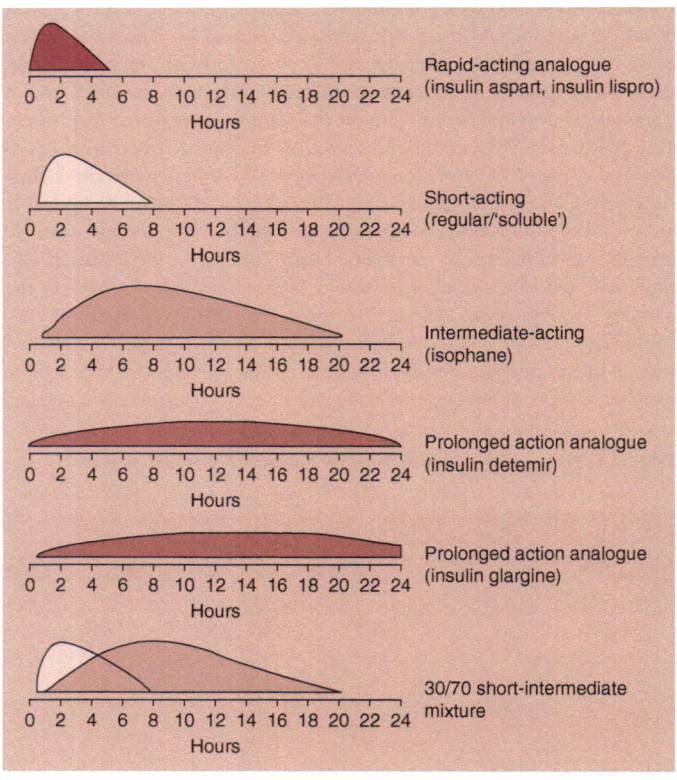

especially hypoglycaemia and weight gain. However, limitations such as day-to-day variability have not been eliminated.

8.2 Ultra-long insulin analogues

Insulin degludec, which has a duration of action of approximately 40 hours (Table 2.5), was approved in Japan in late 2012. The committee for Medicinal Products for Human Use (CHMP) adopted a positive opinion shortly afterwards. Trials in type 2 diabetes have shown a lower risk of nocturnal hypoglycaemia compared with other basal analogues at similar levels of glycaemic control.

Despite these advances in basal therapy insulin is often unduly delayed partly due to negative perceptions of patients and physicians. Arguments for the earlier use of insulin include:

1. The attainment and maintenance of glycaemic control is associated with better long-term clinical outcomes.
2. Early intensive insulin therapy in patients with newly diagnosed type 2 diabetes may have favourable effects on β-cell function and can provide protracted glycaemic remission compared with oral glucose-lowering agents.
3. The risk of severe hypoglycaemia, a major barrier to metabolic control, increases as insulin deficiency becomes more pronounced.
4. Strategies for minimising weight gain during the intensification of treatment are now available.
5. The introduction of insulin treatment does not necessarily impair quality of life. Patients often derive symptomatic benefit as hyperglycaemia is brought under control; the concomitant reduction in pill burden is usually welcomed.
6. Modern delivery devices have eased the inconveniences of insulin therapy; innovations such as pulmonary delivery may offer the prospect of greater acceptability.

Clinical judgement and expertise are prerequisites for success. Recent clinical trials have provided some useful information on strategies for initiating insulin in patients with type 2 diabetes (Box 2.4). Translating the results of clinical trials designed and conducted by experts into routine practice within a primary care setting is, however, a formidable challenge. Chapter 4 contains further details of initiating and monitoring insulin therapy.

8.3 Initiating once-daily insulin

A once-daily injection, usually a small dose pre-bed, e.g. 10 U, is added to oral glucose-lowering therapy. The dose is up-titrated according to fasting blood glucose measurements. Algorithms are available that are generally safe and effective. Prolonged duration insulin analogues, insulin glargine and insulin detemir, are often favoured because of their pharmacokinetic advantages. Insulin analogues provide similar glycaemic control to isophane but with a lower risk of minor hypoglycaemia, notably nocturnally. Insulin analogues are more expensive than isophane insulin but are widely used in the UK.

8.4 Preprandial insulin

This approach, which is popular in some countries, targets postprandial hyperglycaemia, but may be associated with greater weight gain and

> **Box 2.4: Comparison of biphasic, basal, or prandial insulin regimens in patients with type 2 diabetes. Systematic review and meta-analysis of clinical trials using each regimen**
>
> - *Compared with basal insulin, reductions in HbA_{1c} were greater – 0.45% for each – with biphasic and prandial insulin. Reductions in fasting glucose were less with the latter regimen.*
> - *Larger insulin doses were reported for biphasic and prandial regimens compared with basal insulin.*
> - *No differences in major hypoglycaemic events were observed.*
> - *Minor hypoglycaemic events for prandial and biphasic insulin were reported as either higher than or equivalent to basal insulin.*
> - *Greater weight gain – approaching 2 kg – was seen with prandial compared with basal insulin.*
>
> *Data from Lasserson et al. (2009)*

more frequent hypoglycaemia compared with once-daily basal insulin. The 4-T (Treat to Target in Type 2 Diabetes Trial), which compared three regimens of analogue insulin preparations, demonstrated these limitations. In practice, a balanced approach is required that addresses fasting and postprandial glucose control if glycaemic goals are to be attained.

8.5 Basal-bolus regimens

A once or twice-daily prolonged insulin analogue is combined with pre-meal boluses of a rapid-acting insulin analogue. This approach offers flexibility but demands more frequent self-monitoring of blood glucose.

8.6 Premixed biphasic insulin

This may be initiated twice a day, before breakfast and dinner. Premixed, fixed-dose analogue preparations offer the advantage of immediate injection before, or even just after, a meal. In contrast, human sequence or animal derived biphasic insulin preparations should be injected approximately 30–45 min before meals because of the less rapid increase in plasma insulin concentrations. However, some data suggest this may not be necessary and many patients inject just before meals anyway. A third injection is possible using licensed biphasic preparations. High mix insulin formulations that have a greater proportion of rapid-acting insulin have been explored in clinical trials.

8.7 Continuous subcutaneous insulin infusion

This may be a helpful alternative to multiple daily injections in some patients. A comprehensive insulin pump clinical service is required to deliver safe and effective treatment.

8.8 Combined insulin–oral agent strategies

In the absence of any convincing evidence to date that the natural history of type 2 diabetes can be substantially modified by pharmacotherapy, insulin will remain a major – and inevitable – treatment option. Combining insulin with certain DPP-4 inhibitors, glucagon-like peptide 1 mimetics and perhaps other agents currently in development is expanding, although not all drugs in these classes are licensed for use concurrently with insulin. Reductions in body weight and lower insulin doses may be achieved in some patients. Pioglitazone has a licence for use in combination with insulin. This approach may reduce the dose of insulin required in obese patients who often require very large doses of insulin. Definitions of insulin resistance are not particularly helpful in clinical practice, but the scenario in which several hundreds of units of insulin per day appear to be having little impact has become commonplace in the UK. Strategies to counter this impasse are limited.

Combining insulin with metformin, and to a lesser extent pioglitazone, has become routine practice. Several studies have demonstrated the utility of metformin plus insulin combinations; impressive data from clinical trials that show improved glycaemic control with less weight gain and lower rates of hypoglycaemia are not always reproducible in day-to-day practice. The usual approach is to continue metformin when insulin is started, withdrawing drugs such as sulphonylureas.

8.9 Strategies to counter insulin resistance

Obese patients with inadequately controlled type 2 diabetes and those with additional causes of insulin resistance have higher insulin requirements. The use of U500 insulin reduces the volume of each injection. High-strength insulin must be obtained directly from the manufacturer; it is not licensed in the UK. Although formulated as soluble insulin, the pharmacokinetics of U500 insulin resemble those of isophane insulin. Care should be exercised when using insulin in combination with pioglitazone; the risks of weight gain and fluid retention are increased. Insulin clearance is impaired by complications such as renal impairment or the presence of hepatic cirrhosis. Co-administration of metformin or a GLP-1 agonists may be useful.

8.10 Insulin and cancer risk

A series of reports from retrospective studies raised concerns about a potential association between insulin treatment and cancer. Insulin glargine has come under particular scrutiny, but the controversy has not been limited to this analogue. Aspects of the data are conflicting and the interpretation of these reports is potentially open to confounding. An increased risk of cancer is a recognised hazard of obesity even in the absence of diabetes. Another potential confounder is the association between type 2 diabetes per se and colon, pancreas and postmenopausal breast cancer. Closely associated metabolic defects, i.e. insulin resistance and glucose intolerance, have also been linked to some forms of cancer. All of these conditions are characterised by hyper-insulinaemia. An alternative hypothesis, based on epidemiological associations between higher HbA_{1c} levels and cancer, proposes that insulin therapy might be protective via reductions in oxidative stress and other mechanisms. Clinical registry data have provided some support for this possibility.

Evidence of a dose–effect association between insulin treatment and cancer risk has been described. In this context it is noteworthy that epidemiological evidence suggests that metformin, which lowers plasma insulin concentrations, may offer protection against certain forms of cancer. To complicate the picture even further, other classes of diabetes drugs, i.e. GLP-1 receptor agonists, pioglitazone and dapagliflozin (See Chapter 4) have been associated with an increased risk of certain forms of cancer. More data are required and, once again, confounding factors are difficult to exclude. It has been hypothesised that the growth of early tumours might be accelerated by insulin, although the cellular mechanisms are uncertain. Reports of increased affinity of insulin glargine for the insulin-like growth factor-1 receptor in vitro are of uncertain clinical significance. The major metabolites of glargine bind to this receptor with affinities similar to that of human insulin. Additional support for a potentially causal insulin–cancer link comes from the unsettling history of a rapid-acting insulin analogue – B10Asp. The development of this analogue was terminated when evidence of carcinogenicity emerged in preclinical studies. In this case, mammary tumours in rodents were in-creased after exposure to high doses. In contrast, it is apposite to note that insulin detemir exhibits lower mitotic activity *in vitro* compared with human insulin. Thus, molecule-specific effects may be important.

Whereas such observations could provide a prima facie case for a casual association between insulin treatment and cancer no definitive data are available. The general consensus of expert groups is that the evidence is insufficient to warrant any changes in clinical practice, although the European Association for the Study of Diabetes suggested that alternatives to insulin glargine may be considered. Diabetes UK cautioned that the research claiming a link between certain insulins and some cancers should be regarded as inconclusive; patients were advised to continue medication as prescribed and to discuss any concerns with their healthcare team. The response of the EMA was that a causal association between insulin glargine and cancer could not be confirmed or excluded. The results of a large clinical trial (ORIGIN; Outcome Reduction with an Initial Glargine Intervention) published in 2012 provided some reassurance about the safety of glargine in terms of cancer risk. Over a median of 6.2 years follow-up no excess of any form of cancer was observed in subjects with dysglycaemia or type 2 diabetes treated with this insulin analogue.

9. Weight-reducing drugs

The blood glucose-lowering efficacy of lifestyle measures that reduce adiposity in patients with type 2 diabetes is well established. The difficulties faced in achieving and maintaining significant weight loss are, however, readily apparent in daily practice. The history of weight-reducing drugs could perhaps be summarised thus: generally limited efficacy punctuated by periodic safety concerns, compounded by limited tolerability and low concordance rates. The issue of high dropout rates in clinical trials, which can be 30–40%, hampers the interpretation of the efficacy of new agents.

The intestinal lipase inhibitor orlistat 120 mg three times a day with meals can reduce dietary fat absorption by up to 30%. In the context of a reduced fat diet this typically increases weight reduction by an extra 2–3 kg in overweight and obese patients; additional reductions in HbA_{1c} have been reported that are generally lower than those achieved using oral glucose-lowering drugs.

The satiety-inducing serotonin-noradrenaline reuptake inhibitor sibutramine often enables slightly greater reductions of body weight in overweight and obese patients, with extra reductions in HbA_{1c} of approximately 0.5%. Concerns about increases in heart rate and blood pressure in some patients suggested a potential for harm. In 2009, the EMA issued a reminder to prescribers and patients that sibutramine should be used with caution in patients with cardiovascular disease. This was followed in early 2010 by the suspension of marketing authorisation for the drug in the light of an interim analysis of a large post-approval safety trial – the SCOUT (Sibutramine Cardiovascular OUTcomes) study. An excess of cardiovascular events was observed in patients receiving the drug compared with placebo. Of note, the trial included higher-risk patients who would not normally have been candidates for sibutramine. The US Food and Drug Administration took a different line, demanding new warnings about the cardiovascular safety of the drug pending further review of the data.

The first in a new class of agents with beneficial effects on glucose and lipid metabolism, the selective cannabinoid receptor 1 antagonist rimonabant was withdrawn because of concerns about psychological side-effects, including depression with suicidal ideation. In 2012 two new weight-reducing drugs were approved for use in the US. One combines two established drugs: phenteramine + controlled-release topiramate. The other agent - lorcaserin, a serotonin 2C receptor activator - was the first new class of obesity drug to be approved in more than a decade.

Further reading

Ashcroft FM, Gribble FM. ATP-sensitive K+ channels and insulin secretion: their role in health and disease. *Diabetologia.* 1999;42:903-19.

Bailey CJ, Turner RC. Metformin. *N Engl J Med.* 1996;334:574-9.

Bailey CJ, Krentz AJ. Oral Antidiabetic Agents. In: Textbook of Diabetes, 4th edition (Chapter 29). Edited by R. Holt, B. Goldstein, A. Flyvbjerg and C. Cockram. London: Wiley Blackwell, 2010: 452–77.

Bailey CJ. Metformin: effects on micro and macrovascular complications in type 2 diabetes. *Cardiovasc Drug Ther.* 2008;22:215-24.

Blickle JF. Meglitinide analogues: a review of clinical data focused on recent trials. *Diabetes Metab.* 2006;32:113-20.

Chiasson JL, Josse RG, Gomis R, et al. Acarbose for the prevention of diabetes mellitus: the STOP–NIDDM randomised trial. STOP–NIDDM Trial Research Group. *Lancet.* 2002;359:2072-7.

Cryer PE. Diverse causes of hypoglycaemia-associated autonomic failure in diabetes. *N Engl J Med.* 2004;350:2272-9.

Cusi K, DeFronzo RA. Metformin: a review of its metabolic effects. *Diabetes Rev.* 1998;6: 89-131.

Diabetes Prevention Program Research Group. Reduction of the incidence of type 2 diabetes with lifestyle intervention or metformin. *N Engl J Med.* 2002;346:393-403.

Dormandy J, Charbonnel B, Eckland D, et al. Secondary prevention of macrovascular events in patients with type 2 diabetes in the PROactive study (PROspective pioglitAzone Clinical Trial In macroVascular Events): a randomised controlled trial. *Lancet.* 2005;366:1279-89.

Dornhorst A. Insulotropic meglitinide analogues. *Lancet.* 2001;358:1709-15.

Hermann LS, Lindberg G, Lindblad U, et al. Efficacy, effectiveness and safety of sulphonylurea–metformin combination therapy in patients with type 2 diabetes. *Diabetes Obes Metab.* 2002;4:296-304.

Hermansen K, Mortensen LS. Body weight changes associated with antihyperglycaemic agents in type 2 diabetes mellitus. *Drug Saf.* 2007;30:1127-42.

Hirsch IB. Insulin analogues. *N Engl J Med.* 2005;352:174-83.

Holman RR, Haffner SM, McMurray JJ, et al. Effect of nateglinide on the incidence of diabetes and cardiovascular events. *N Engl J Med.* 2010;362:1463-76.

Holman RR, Paul SK, Bethel MA, et al. 10-Year follow-up of intensive glucose control in type 2 diabetes. *N Engl J Med.* 2008;359:1577-89.

Horvath K, Jeitler K, Berghold A, et al. Long-acting insulin analogues versus NPH insulin (human isophane insulin) for type 2 diabetes mellitus. *Cochrane Database Syst Rev.* 2007;2:CD005613.

Kahn SE, Haffner SM, Heise MA, et al. ADOPT Study Group. Glycemic durability of rosiglitazone, metformin, or glyburide monotherapy. *N Engl J Med.* 2006;355:2427-43.

Krentz AJ. Rosiglitazone: Trials, tribulations and termination. *Drugs.* 2011;71:123-30.

Krentz AJ. Thiazolidinediones: effects on the development and progression of type 2 diabetes and associated vascular complications. *Diabetes Metab Res Rev.* 2009;25:112-26.

Krentz AJ, Bailey CJ. Oral antidiabetic agents: current role in type 2 diabetes mellitus. *Drugs*. 2005;65:385-411.

Krentz AJ, Ferner RE, Bailey CJ. Comparative tolerability profiles of oral antidiabetic agents. *Drug Saf*. 1994;11:223-41.

Lamanna C, Monami M, Marchionni N, et al. Effects of metformin on cardiovascular effects and mortality: a meta-analysis of randomized clinical trials. *Diabetes Obes Metab* 2011;13:221-8

Lasserson DS, Glasziou P, Perera R, et al. Optimal insulin regimens in type 2 diabetes: systematic review and meta-analyses. *Diabetologia* 2009;52:1990-2000

Lloret-Linares C, Greenfield JR, Czernichow S. Effects of weight-reducing agents on glycaemic parameters and progression to type 2 diabetes: a review. *Diabetic Med*. 2008;25: 1142-50.

McGuire DK, Inzucchi SE. New drugs for the treatment of diabetes mellitus. Part 1. Thiazolidinediones and their evolving cardiovascular implications. *Circulation*. 2008;117(3): 440-9.

Nesto RW, Bell D, Bonow RO, et al. Thiazolidinedione use, fluid retention, and congestive heart failure: a consensus statement from the American Heart Association and the American Diabetes Association. *Circulation*. 2003;108:2941-8.

Nissen SE, Wolski K. Effect of rosiglitazone on the risk of myocardial infarction and death from cardiovascular causes. *N Engl J Med*. 2007;356:2457-71.

Smith U, Gale EA. Does diabetes therapy influence the risk of cancer? *Diabetologia*. 2009;52: 1699-708.

Rao AD, Kuhadiya N, Reynolds K, Fonseca VA. Is the combination of sulphonylureas and metformin associated with an increased risk of cardiovascular disease or all-cause mortality?: a meta-analysis of observational studies. *Diabetes Care*. 2008;31:1672-8.

Rucker D, Padwal R, Li SK, et al. Long term pharmacotherapy for obesity and overweight: updated meta-analysis. *BMJ*. 2007;335:1194-99.

The ORIGIN Trial Investigators. Basal insulin and cardiovascular and other outcomes in dysglycemia. *N Engl J Med*. 2012 (10.1056/NEJMoa1203858).

Woodcock J, Sharfstein JM, Hamburg M. Regulatory action on rosiglitazone by the U.S. Food and Drug Administration. *N Engl J Med*. 2010;363:1489-91.

Wang F, Surh J, Kaur M. Insulin degludec as an ultralong-acting basal insulin once a day: a systematic review. *Diabetes Metab Syndr Obes*. 2012;5:191-204.

Weng J, Li Y, Xu W, et al. Effect of intensive insulin therapy on beta-cell function and glycaemic control in patients with newly diagnosed type 2 diabetes: a multicentre randomised parallel-group trial. *Lancet*. 2008;371:1753-60.

Yki-Jarvinen H. Combination therapies with insulin in type 2 diabetes. *Diabetes Care*. 2001;24:758-67.

Yki-Jarvinen H. Thiazolidinediones. *N Engl J Med*. 2004;351:1106-18.

Chapter 3

Recently introduced and emerging classes of glucose-lowering drugs

1. Drugs acting on the incretin system

Insulin secretagogues such as sulphonylureas cause insulin release irrespective of the prevailing glucose concentration. Enhancing insulin secretion through a glucose-dependent mechanism is an attractive, novel therapeutic approach that can circumvent some of the unwanted effects of sulphonylureas – principally weight gain and hypoglycaemia. This approach would be expected to restore the defective β-cell insulin secretion pathway without causing excessive hyperinsulinaemia and carry an intrinsically lower risk of iatrogenic hypoglycaemia. In recent years, novel drugs have become available that are designed to fulfill these aims.

2. Pathophysiology of the incretin system in type 2 diabetes

Gastrointestinal polypeptide hormones secreted in response to the ingestion of a meal augment insulin secretion; this is known as the incretin effect and is held to account for up to 70% of postprandial insulin secretion (Figure 3.1). The most important incretins are glucagon-like peptide (GLP)-1 and glucose-dependent insulinotropic polypeptide (GIP). These hormones are secreted by the L cells of the distal ileum and colon, and the K cells of the duodenum and upper jejunum, respectively. Circulating levels rise within minutes of eating, implying likely stimulation by neuroendocrine pathways. Incretin hormones act by means of specific β-cell G-protein-coupled receptors to enhance glucose-stimulated insulin secretion. The acute effect of GLP-1 on β cells is the stimulation of glucose-dependent insulin release; this is followed by enhancement of insulin biosynthesis and stimulation of transcription of the insulin gene.

The incretin effect is deficient in patients with type 2 diabetes, mainly because of reduced postprandial GLP-1 secretion (see Figure 3.1). Reduced GLP-1 levels are accompanied by a reduced insulinotropic action of GIP. The cause of these defects is presently unclear. GLP-1, but not GIP, slows gastric emptying and also suppresses appetite, effects that are impaired by deficiency of the hormone in type 2 diabetes.

There is abundant experimental evidence that inappropriate glucagon secretion plays a role in the development of hyperglycaemia in type 2 diabetes, sustaining hepatic glucose production rates in the presence of relative insulin deficiency; this defect in islet α-cell function is thought to

A. J. Krentz, *Drug Therapy for Type 2 Diabetes*
DOI: 10.1007/978-1-908517-77-7_3,
© Springer International Publishing Switzerland 2012

Figure 3.1. The incretin effect.

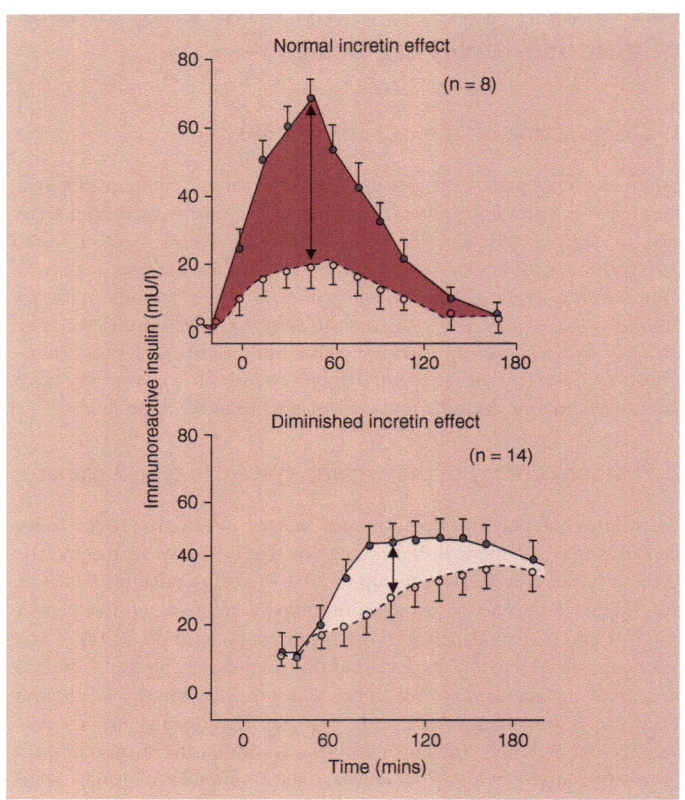

○——○ Intravenous glucose infusion; ●——● oral glucose load.

The incretin effect is diminished in type 2 diabetes. In the top panel insulin secretion is greater when glucose is given orally, compared to matched blood glucose levels achieved by intravenous infusion. The enhanced response is known as the incretin effect. In the lower panel the insulin response to oral glucose is smaller and less rapidly achieved in subjects with type 2 diabetes: this reflects reduced activity of the incretin axis in type 2 diabetes.

Data from Nauck et al. (1986).

reflect impaired cellular glucose sensing. GLP-1 suppresses glucagon secretion during hyperglycaemia. The counterregulatory secretion of glucagon in response to hypoglycaemia, however, is preserved even in the presence of pharmacological concentrations of GLP-1. Inappropriate glucagon secretion is reduced by the incretin system (Table 3.1).

Studies in rodents and human islets indicate that GLP-1 can promote the expansion of β-cell mass. To date, however, there is no convincing evidence that this effect is reproduced in humans with type 2 diabetes. In addition to islet β and α cells the tissue distribution of the GLP-1 receptor includes the central and peripheral nervous system, kidney, lung and gastrointestinal tract. GLP-1 receptors are also present in the myocardium where their stimulation reduces ischaemic injury in animal models.

GLP-1 and GIP are subject to rapid degradation mainly by a ubiquitous cell surface enzyme dipeptidyl peptidase (DPP)-4, which cleaves two N-terminal amino acids thereby removing insulinotropic activity. The half-life of GLP-1 in the circulation is less than 2 min, and ~7 min for GIP. Numerous gastrointestinal hormones, cytokines and chemopeptides are also substrates for DPP-4. The enzyme, which is a member of a wider family, is also the CD26 T-cell-activating antigen found in nearly all human tissues.

Novel therapies that exploit the incretin effect of GLP-1 include the orally active DPP-4 inhibitors and the injectable GLP mimetics. The latter fall into two categories: (1) derivatives of GLP-1 modified to resist proteolysis and (2) novel peptides that have metabolic actions similar to GLP-1 and are intrinsically resistant to proteolysis. The GLP-1 receptor agonists licensed in the UK are exenatide (twice-daily and once-weekly formulations) and liraglutide. The place of these agents in treatment algorithms is being explored.

3. Dipeptidyl peptidase 4 inhibitors

DPP-4 inhibitors, also known as gliptins, enhance the levels of the intestinally secreted incretins GLP-1 and GIP through selective inhibition of the enzyme DPP-4 (Figure 3.2). Drugs in this class are now being incorporated into management pathways for type 2 diabetes. Sitagliptin and vildagliptin were introduced in the UK in 2007 and 2008, respectively. Saxagliptin is available in the USA, and received marketing authorisation

Table 3.1. Effects of the incretin hormones GLP-1 and GIP on glucose homeostasis reported in clinical studies.

	GLP-1	GIP
Effects on pancreatic islets		
Increase nutrient-induced insulin secretion	Y	Y
Suppress glucagon secretion	Y	–
Increase somatostatin secretion	Y	–
Extra-pancreatic effects		
Slow gastric emptying	Y	–
Promote satiety and weight reduction	Y	–
Promote lipogenesis	–	Y

GIP: Glucose-dependent insulinotropic polypeptide; GLP-1: glucagon-like peptide-1.

in the European Union in 2009. The drugs differ in their metabolism and safety profiles (Table 3.2). Sitagliptin is currently available in three fixed-dose combinations with metformin: 50/500 mg, 50/850 mg and 50/1000 mg. Vildagliptin is offered as fixed-dose combinations with metformin: 50/850 mg and 50/1000 mg. In the USA, the Food and Drug Administration (FDA) demanded additional clinical safety data before it could approve vildagliptin. This followed evidence of skin lesions in a primate model and issues of safety in patients with renal impairment.

In 2011, the FDA and EMA approved linagliptin, which has a primarily non-renal route of elimination (see below). Linagliptin has been approved for combination with insulin as well as in combination with certain oral glucose-lowering agents. Other DPP-4 inhibitors are in development, including alogliptin, for which the results of further safety and efficacy studies are awaited.

3.1 Pharmacokinetics

Sitagliptin, vildagliptin and saxagliptin are selective, competitive, reversible inhibitors of DPP-4. Sitagliptin is non-covalently bound to DPP-4, whereas vildagliptin and saxagliptin bind covalently. Selectivity of action has been an important consideration in the development of these drugs. For sitagliptin, no inhibition of DPP-8 and DPP-9, gene members of the S9b family of dipeptidyl peptidases, is anticipated at exposures required for glucose lowering in humans.

Sitagliptin – This has high bioavailability (~90%) and a plasma half-life of 8–14 h; T_{max} is 1–4 h. Plasma protein binding is relatively low at approximately 40%. A small proportion of the drug is hepatically metabolised by CYP3A4 and CYP2C6. Approximately 80% of sitagliptin is eliminated unchanged in the urine through renal tubular secretion. A single dose of 100 mg sitagliptin achieves near complete inhibition of DPP-4 activity for approximately 12 h, with >95% inhibition up to 24 h.

Figure 3.2. Effect of dipeptidyl peptidase 4 (DPP-4) inhibitors on glucagon-like peptide 1 (GLP-1) metabolism and its physiological actions.

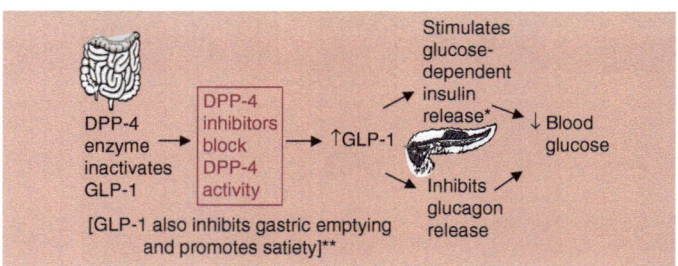

*And gene expression in animal models.

**DPP-4 inhibition does not lead to clinically significant effects in patients with type 2 diabetes.

Vildagliptin – This has a shorter plasma half-life: 1.5–4.5 h. T_{max} is less than 2 h. Bioavailability is approximately 85%. The majority of vildagliptin (~70%) undergoes predominantly renal metabolism to inactive metabolites with a negligible contribution from CYP450 isoforms; most (~85%) is eliminated in the urine. A dose of 50–100 mg vildagliptin will provide almost complete inhibition of DPP-4 for approximately 12 h and approximately 40% inhibition at 24 h. Plasma protein binding is less than 10%.

Saxagliptin – Maximal inhibition of DPP-4 occurs 2–3 h after oral administration; the suppression of DPP-4 activity extends to 24 h. Saxagliptin is eliminated by both renal and hepatic pathways. Hepatic metabolism creates a hydroxylated metabolite that has approximately 50% of the activity of the parent compound. There is evidence of active renal excretion of the parent compound. Circulating levels of saxagliptin and its metabolite are increased by renal impairment. *In vitro* serum protein binding is 30% or less in humans.

3.2 Clinical applications

In principle, DPP-4 inhibitors can be used as monotherapy in patients with type 2 diabetes who have responded inadequately to lifestyle measures. This is not, however, permitted in all countries. At present, DPP-4 inhibitors tend to be preferred as second or third-line therapy in patients inadequately controlled by metformin, a sulphonylurea, or a thiazolidinedione. Theoretically, they could be used with any other class of oral agent or insulin, as their mode of action on the β cell is different to that of sulphonylureas and meglitinides; moreover, their ability to reduce glucagon levels may provide a useful adjunct to insulin therapy even when there is major β-cell dysfunction. In the UK, sitaglipitin is approved for addition to a stable dose of insulin, with or without metformin. Improvements in β-cell function reflect the mode of action of the drugs and are dependent on β-cell reserves. The absence of weight-promoting actions makes the DPP-4 inhibitors especially suitable for overweight and obese patients. The low intrinsic risk of hypoglycaemia when used in conjunction with non-insulin-releasing agents makes them suitable for higher-risk groups. These include individuals who are already approaching glycaemic targets, or have unpredictable meal patterns.

Sitagliptin 100 mg is required once a day and can be taken with or without food; vildagliptin 50 mg is usually taken twice a day. Lower dosages are recommended if combined with a sulphonylurea. In the UK the licence for sitagliptin includes monotherapy if metformin cannot be used; in combination with a sulphonylurea; in combination with a thiazolidinedione (pioglitazone); in combination with metformin plus sulphonylurea; and in combination with metformin plus thiazolidinedione. Sitagliptin is also approved in the UK as add-on to insulin, or insulin and metformin.

Table 3.2. Dosages and precautions of DPP-4 inhibitors.

	Usual dose	Liver disease	Renal disease	Other comments
Sitagliptin	100 mg/day	May be used in mild-to-moderate liver disease, i.e. Child–Pugh score 7–9 (a composite of biochemical and clinical criteria)	Not recommended in moderate to severe renal failure.*	Reports of pancreatitis; causality not confirmed
Vildagliptin	50 mg twice a day	Avoid if serum transaminase levels elevated ×3 or more before or during therapy	Not recommended if creatinine clearance <50 ml/min	Check liver function before initiation, every 3 months during first year of treatment and periodically thereafter
Saxagliptin	5 mg/day	No dose reduction required	Use 2.5 mg daily with moderate or severe renal impairment (i.e. creatinine clearance ≥30 to <50 ml/min). Not recommended in severe renal failure requiring haemodialysis.	

DPP-4: Dipeptidyl peptidase 4.
* NB. Recommendations differ between countries.

Saxagliptin is usually taken once a day in a dose of 5 mg. The dose of saxagliptin should be reduced to 2.5 mg once daily and used with caution in patients with moderate or severe renal impairment (i.e. creatinine clearance ≥30 to <50 ml/min). Saxagliptin is not recommended for patients with end-stage renal disease requiring haemodialysis. The UK licence includes use with metformin, a sulphonylurea if metformin is inappropriate, and with a thiazolidinedione; in all these situations diet and exercise will have been deemed to be providing inadequate glycaemic control.

Vildagliptin is licensed in the UK for use as dual oral therapy in combination with metformin, in patients with insufficient glycaemic control despite the maximal tolerated dose of monotherapy with metformin; with a sulphonylurea, in patients with insufficient glycaemic control despite the maximal tolerated dose of a sulphonylurea and for whom metformin is inappropriate due to contraindications or intolerance; and a thiazolidinedione, in patients with insufficient glycaemic control. In 2012 approval was recommended for use of vildagliptin in combination with insulin by the EMA.

The glucose-dependent action of these agents reduces the risk of excessive reductions in blood glucose, unless combined with a sulphonylurea. There is thus no dose titration. Monitoring of fasting and postprandial glycaemia aids assessment of response. If hypoglycaemia occurs when a DPP-4 inhibitor is combined with a sulphonylurea, reducing the dose of the sulphonylurea or withdrawal of the DPP-4 inhibitor is recommended.

3.3 Cautions and contraindications

Sitagliptin is mainly eliminated unchanged in the urine. In the USA, a reduced dose is recommended for patients with moderate renal insufficiency, i.e. creatinine clearance of 30 ml/min or more to less than 50 ml/min; for patients with severe renal insufficiency or with end-stage renal disease requiring haemodialysis or peritoneal dialysis, a dose of 25 mg once a day should be considered. Sitagliptin does not appear to affect P450 isoforms; this allows its use in patients with minor to moderate impairment of liver function, provided renal function is adequate. The levels of saxagliptin and its active metabolite are reduced in patients with impaired hepatic function. The dose of saxagliptin should be reduced to 2.5 mg once daily in patients with moderate or severe renal impairment. In view of the renal metabolism and elimination of vildagliptin, its use is not recommended in patients with moderate or severe renal impairment. The primarily non-renal route of elimination of linagliptin means that no dose reduction is required in patients with renal impairment. Some cases of reversible elevations in alanine aminotransferase or aspartate aminotransferase have been observed in patients receiving vildagliptin. Clinical chemistry assessment of liver function is recommended before starting treatment, at 3-month intervals in the first year, and periodically thereafter. A marked rise in liver enzymes, e.g. alanine aminotransferase or aspartate aminotransferase more than three times the upper limit of the normal range, or other signs of hepatic impairment contraindicate continued treatment. No significant drug interactions have been noted with sitagliptin, vildagliptin, or saxagliptin. DPP-4 inhibitors should be avoided in women planning conception and during pregnancy.

Saxagliptin is being evaluated in a cardiovascular outcomes study to fulfill a US FDA postmarketing requirement. No evidence of cardiovascular risk has emerged to date. A pooled analysis of phase IIb and III trials suggested a trend towards a reduction in cardiovascular events compared with placebo or active comparators.

3.4 Efficacy

Sitagliptin – In clinical trials, the administration of 100 mg/day sitagliptin as monotherapy or add-on therapy to other oral agents typically reduced glycated haemoglobin (HbA_{1c}) from a baseline of approximately 8% by approximately 0.7 percentage points after 24–52 weeks. Individuals with higher baseline HbA_{1c} levels have shown reductions in HbA_{1c} greater than 1%; this observation, i.e. greater glucose lowering with higher baseline HbA_{1c} levels, is not unique to this class of agents. Fasting plasma glucose concentrations were reduced by approximately 1.0–1.5 mmol/l, and postprandial glucose levels measured 2 h after a standard mixed meal were usually reduced by approximately 3 mmol/l. Sitagliptin did not cause a clinically significant increase in the incidence of hypoglycaemia; the combination of sitagliptin plus metformin was associated with fewer espisodes of hypoglycaemia than a combination of glipizide plus metformin at similar levels of HbA_{1c} reduction. Sitagliptin did not increase body weight compared with placebo in clinical trials.

Vildagliptin – In trials, a single daily dose of 50–100 mg/day vildagliptin showed similar efficacy and tolerability to sitagliptin when used as monotherapy or as add-on therapy to metformin or a thiazolidinedione. The dose of vildagliptin should be 50 mg once a day when combined with a sulphonylurea. Several trials with vildagliptin produced slightly greater reductions in HbA_{1c}, but these tended to be associated with slightly higher average baseline HbA_{1c} levels, i.e. greater than 8.5%. There was no increase in hypoglycaemia or changes in mean body weight with vildagliptin.

Saxaglipitin – In clinical trials, a dose of 5 mg a day either as monotherapy, or in combination with metformin, a sulphonylurea, or a thiazolidinedione produced mean placebo-subtracted reductions in HbA_{1c} in the range of approximately 0.60–0.65%. No excess of hypoglycaemia or weight gain was observed in phase III trials compared with placebo.

3.5 Adverse effects

To date no serious adverse effects have been reported. Unlike GLP-1 agonists, upper gastrointestinal side-effects are not a feature of DPP-4 therapy. In clinical trials generally of 6–12 months' duration, tolerability and adverse events were broadly similar to placebo or the comparator drug, although there have been reports of higher rates of nasopharyngitis and upper respiratory tract infections. The aforementioned increases in liver enzymes observed with the 100 mg dose of vildagliptin does not appear to be relevant to the 50 mg dose that is marketed.

The many natural substrates for DPP-4 include a range of cytokines and chemokines. The theoretical impact of the drugs on these peptides needs to be borne in mind as patients become exposed to the long-term inhibition of DPP-4. The increased frequency of upper respiratory tract infections, less than 5% in trials, gives pause for thought about the potential for interference with innate immune protection and lymphocyte activation antigen. Neither CD26 knockout mice nor the DPP-4-specific inhibitors used in animals or humans have shown any significant untoward immune-related effects to date. Minor decreases in the blood lymphocyte count have been observed with saxagliptin.

The importance of selective DPP-4 inhibition is suggested by the observation that the inhibition of related enzymes such as DPP-8 and DPP-9 has produced blood dyscrasias and cutaneous lesions in some species; however, this toxicity has not been encountered in clinical use.

In 2009, the FDA notified healthcare professionals and patients of revisions to the prescribing information for sitagliptin and sitagliptin/metformin to include reports of acute pancreatitis. It is recommended that patients be monitored carefully for the development of pancreatitis after the initiation or dose increases. Sitagliptin should be used with caution in patients with a history of pancreatitis. No clear cause-effect association has been identified.

4. Glucagon-like peptide 1 agonists

GLP-1 receptor agonists mimic the actions of endogenous GLP-1 at its cellular receptor. At therapeutic plasma concentrations exenatide has the capacity to restore the first-phase insulin response to an intravenous bolus of glucose in patients with type 2 diabetes; second-phase insulin secretion is also increased. Thus, the main glucose-lowering effect occurs in the postprandial period. Drugs in this class are designed to be resistant to the actions of DPP-4. The mode of action of GLP-1 agonists is reminiscent of normal physiology insofar that they induce insulin secretion in a glucose-dependent fashion. However, they are potent pharmacological agents. Their effects on insulin secretion (increased) and glucagon secretion (decreased), gastric emptying rate (slowed) and satiety (enhanced) are well documented. The effect on gastric emptying brings problems of nausea and vomiting that often accompany the initiation of GLP-1 receptor agonists. Compared with the orally active DPP-4 inhibitors, GLP-1 agonists generally offer greater reductions in glucose allied to variable decreases in body weight. Calorie intake tends to be reduced. At first sight these are desirable effects that have generated considerable enthusiasm. Indeed, weight loss in the context of improved glycaemic control fills a much-needed gap in therapy. Given the limited experience with GLP-1 agonists, however, a cautious approach to their use seems sensible. The long-term effects of pharmacological stimulation of the widely distributed GLP-1 receptor are not known. Whereas β-cell function is improved by GLP-1 receptor agonists, evidence that this translates into a sustained effect that provides a clinically significant advantage over other therapies is not yet available. The effects of exenatide on measures of β-cell function, which sit in contrast to insulin therapy as a comparator, have generated interest in using GLP-1 agonists as first-line pharmacotherapy. The rationale of this approach is that the early use of these agents might preserve β-cell function, while acknowledging that this is already severely compromised. It has been hypothesised that the combination of a GLP-1 agonist with a thiazolidinedione might be particularly advantageous. This hypothesis is being tested in clinical trials.

The long-term impact of GLP-1 agonists on clinical outcomes has not been determined. In clinical trials a higher discontinuation rate compared with insulin has been apparent with GLP-1 receptor agonists. Some physicians use GLP-1 receptor agonists to reduce insulin doses and limit weight gain in the knowledge that this is currently an unlicensed indication. Other GLP-1 receptor agonists that require less frequent administration are in development, including taspoglutide, lixisenatide and albiglutide. However, in 2011 phase III trials of taspoglutide were suspended because of issues of hypersensitivity and gastrointestinal intolerance.

4.1 Exenatide

Synthetic exendin-4, known as exenatide, was approved for use in the USA in 2005; it has been available in the UK since 2007. Exendin-4 is a homologue of GLP-1 that was discovered in the venom of *Heloderma suspectum*, otherwise known as the Gila monster, a lizard native to the southwestern USA and northern Mexico. The resistance to inactivation of a DDP-4 provided the rationale for the development of exenatide. Liraglutide was approved in 2009. GLP-1 mimetics lower HbA_{1c} approximately 1% compared with placebo and induced weight loss (~1.5 kg and 4.5–5.0 kg versus placebo and insulin, respectively). Open label extension studies have shown that improvements in glycaemic control can be sustained with progressive reductions in body weight. Benefits in glycaemic control and body weight may be accompanied by favourable changes in blood pressure, lipid profiles and blood hepatic transaminase levels.

4.1.1 Pharmacokinetics

Exenatide has a 53% sequence homology with human GLP-1. The pharmacokinetic profile of the molecule has profound differences to the native hormone. In preclinical studies, exenatide had a 20–30-fold longer half-life and greater than 5000-fold greater glucose-lowering potency than GLP-1. Resistance to inactivation by DDP-4 is achieved by the substitution of Gly2 for Ala2 at the inactivation site of the molecule. Exenatide is regarded as exhibiting dose-proportional kinetics. It is rapidly absorbed, being detectable in the blood within 15 min after subcutaneous injection. Maximum drug concentrations are achieved at approximately 2–3 h. The formation of antibodies can reportedly increase the C_{max} and may lengthen the half-life of the drug. Effects on blood glucose are evident for 6–8 h after injection, hence the need for twice-daily administration. The elimination half-life of exenatide is approximately 3–4 h. Non-clinical studies have shown that exenatide is primarily cleared by the renal system; in human studies clearance and tolerability of the drug are reduced in patients with severe renal impairment.

4.1.2 Clinical applications

In the USA, exenatide is approved as adjunctive therapy for patients with inadequate glycaemic control taking metformin, a sulphonylurea, a thiazolidinedione, a combination of metformin and a sulphonylurea, or a combination of metformin and a thiazolidinedione. In 2011 exenatide was approved by the FDA for use as add-on therapy to insulin glargine. In the UK, exenatide is approved for use with metformin, sulphonylureas or pioglitazone (including certain combinations) in patients who have not achieved adequate glycaemic control on maximally tolerated doses of these agents. Exenatide is also licensed as adjunctive therapy with a basal insulin, with or without metformin and/or pioglitazone.

Insulin secretion is coupled closely to plasma glucose levels so no reduction in the dose of exenatide is necessary for meal size or activity levels, i.e. the dose does not need to be adjusted on a day-by-day basis. Clinical trials show a small but significant risk of hypoglycaemia when exenatide is used in conjunction with a sulphonylurea; self-monitoring of blood glucose may be necessary to adjust the sulphonylurea dose. When added to metformin, no dose adjustment of the oral agent is required. Limited experience exists concerning the combination therapy with thiazolidinediones. Safety considerations in specific patient groups include:

- Elderly patients: exenatide should be used with caution; dose escalation from 5 µg to 10 µg should proceed with care in patients over 70 years. Clinical experience with exenatide in patients over 75 years is very limited.
- Patients with renal impairment: no dosage adjustment is necessary in patients with mild renal impairment, defined as a creatinine clearance of 50–80 ml/min. For a creatinine clearance of 30–50 ml/min, dose escalation from 5 µg to 10 µg should proceed cautiously. Drug-induced nausea and vomiting may produce transient hypovolaemia, thereby compromising renal function. Exenatide is not recommended in patients with severe renal impairment, i.e. creatinine clearance less than 30 ml/min.
- Patients with hepatic impairment: no dosage adjustment is necessary.

Exenatide is administered as a twice-daily subcutaneous injection using a prefilled pen device in the thigh, abdomen, or upper arm. The starting dose is 5 μg given any time within the 60-min period before the morning and evening meal, or before the two main meals of the day approximately 6 h or more apart. The drug should not be administered after meals. The dose is increased to 10 μg twice a day after 4 weeks if tolerated and according to the clinical response. If gastrointestinal side-effects are troublesome, dose escalation can be deferred for a further 4–6 weeks. The currently held view is that weight loss is generally unrelated to drug-induced nausea.

4.1.3 Efficacy and tolerability

Exenatide is associated with reductions in HbA_{1c} of approximately 1%, accompanied by decreases in fasting plasma glucose concentrations, and dose-dependent progressive weight loss compared with placebo. Weight reduction is clinically significant in many patients. Nausea is the most commonly reported side-effect; this is usually judged to be mild and tends to reduce with time. In trials approximately 30–45% of patients experience nausea, vomiting, or diarrhoea; 5–15% of patients discontinue treatment because of side-effects. Although hypoglycaemia may occur when exenatide is administered in combination with a sulphonylurea, this is rarely severe, i.e. it can be self-managed. Similar reductions in HbA_{1c} are associated with weight loss in exenatide-treated patients and weight gain when insulin is used as a comparator. There are no adequate studies of exenatide in pregnancy.

By October 2007, the FDA had received 30 post-marketing reports of acute pancreatitis in patients taking exenatide. Most of the patients had risk factors such as gallstones, severe hypertriglyceridaemia or excessive alcohol use. The FDA requested that the manufacturer change the drug's label to include information about pancreatitis. Physicians should instruct patients taking the drug to seek medical care promptly if they develop symptoms suggestive of pancreatitis. Immediate medical attention should be sought if severe or persistent abdominal pain or persistent severe nausea or vomiting develops. Exenatide should be discontinued if pancreatitis is suspected, and should not be restarted unless an alternative aetiology is identified with confidence.

The long-term clinical significance of antibodies to exenatide, which have been observed in approximately 40% of patients, is uncertain, but the metabolic effects of exenatide may be impaired in the presence of high titres.

Exenatide LAR is a sustained-release formulation of injectable microspheres of the drug and poly(D,L lactic-co-glycolic acid), a biodegradable polymer. Gradual drug delivery at a controlled rate results in exenatide LAR being suitable for once-weekly injection. After 2 weeks of treatment with 2.0 mg exenatide LAR, drug concentrations sufficient to reduce plasma glucose significantly are achieved. At approximately 6 weeks with this dose, plasma exenatide concentrations are similar to the maximum concentration achieved with a single injection of 10 μg exenatide.

The drug has been compared with exenatide in clinical trials. Improved glycaemic control and beneficial effects on body weight have been reported using once-weekly exenatide LAR. In a head-to-head study in obese patients with type 2 diabetes, exenatide LAR reduced levels of HbA_{1c} by almost half a percentage point more than exenatide given twice a day (Figure 3.3A). Both treatments resulted in similar reductions in body weight of just over 3.5 kg at 30 weeks (Figure 3.3B). Reductions in blood pressure were observed in both groups, with greater lowering of cholesterol levels with the once-weekly treatment. Limited data suggest that cardiovascular events may be reduced by twice-daily exenatide. This observation seems consistent with cardio-protective effects of the drug in animal models mediated via GLP-1 receptors on myocardial cells. Local reactions, principally injection site pruritis, were more frequent with exenatide LAR. Neutralising antibodies were associated with a smaller reduction in HbA_{1c}. Extended-release exenatide received a positive recommendation from the EMA in June 2011 for use in combination with metformin, a sulphonylurea, a glitazone, or with metformin plus a sulphonylurea or a glitazone. After requiring electrocardiographic safety data the FDA approved exenatide LAR in 2012.

4.2 Liraglutide

Liraglutide is a DPP-4-resistant GLP-1 mimetic consisting of a modified GLP-1 sequence attached to a palmitoyl chain, which confers an affinity to albumin that enables non-covalent binding to serum albumin following subcutaneous administration.

4.2.1 Pharmacokinetics

Albumin binding delays renal elimination of the drug, giving liraglutide a half-life of approximately 12 h in humans. Liraglutide has a 97% sequence identity to native GLP-1 and is suitable for administration by once-daily injection. The absorption of liraglutide from subcutaneous tissue is slow and reaches maximum concentration after approximately 8–12 h. The avoidance of peaks of plasma drug levels may help to attenuate gastrointestinal side-effects. Two minor metabolites are generated by routes of metabolism similar to those for other large proteins. The elimination half-life of the drug is approximately 13 h. The potential for pharmacokinetic interactions with other drugs by cytochrome P450 is considered low.

4.2.2 Indications and cautions

In the UK, liraglutide was approved in 2010 for the treatment of adults with type 2 diabetes in combination with metformin or a sulphonylurea; in patients with insufficient glycaemic control on the maximal tolerated dose of metformin or sulphonylurea monotherapy; or in combination with metformin and a sulphonylurea; or metformin and a thiazolidinedione in patients with insufficient glycaemic control on dual therapy. In the USA,

Figure 3.3. Efficacy of exenatide once weekly versus twice daily. (A) Change in HbA$_{1c}$ from baseline over 30 weeks (least square mean [SE], intention-to-treat population, n = 295). Baseline HbA$_{1c}$ values were 8.3% (SD 1.0 for both ex-enatide arms. Greater reductions in HbA$_{1c}$ with exenatide once a week versus twice a day were significant from week 10 (p < 0.01); HbA$_{1c}$ changes at endpoint were -1.9% (0.08) and -1.5% (0.08; p = 0.023). **(B)** Change in bodyweight from baseline over 30 weeks (least square mean [SE], intention-to-treat population, n = 295). Similar reductions in bodyweight were shown with exenatide once a week (3.7 [0.5] kg) and twice a day (3.6 [0.5] kg).

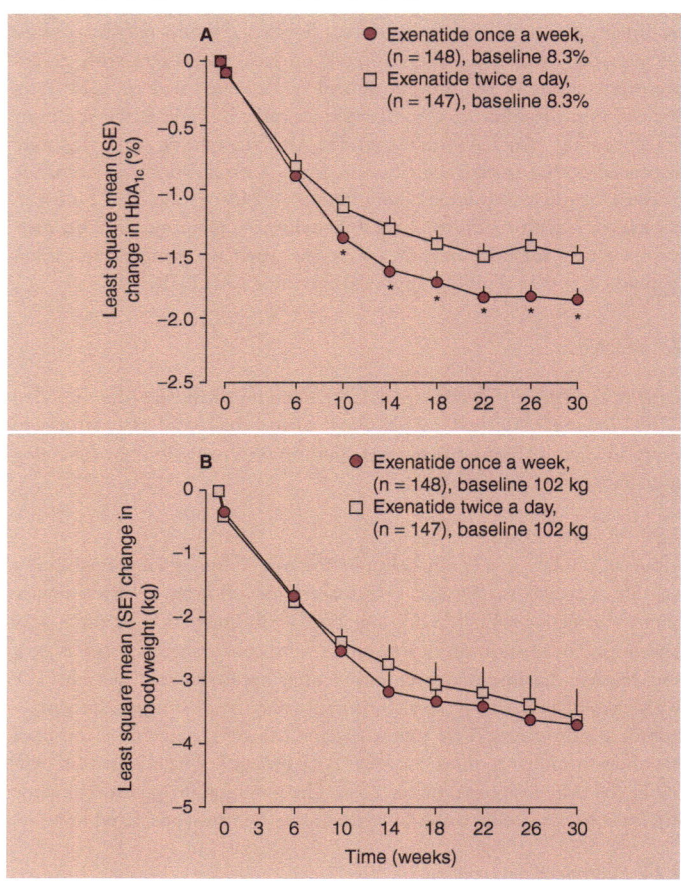

Reproduced from Drucker et al. (2008), with permission.

liraglutide was approved in 2010 for use in conjunction with diet and exercise to improve glycaemic control in adults with type 2 diabetes either as monotherapy or in combination with other glucose-lowering medications.

The FDA stipulated post-marketing safety studies: first, a 5-year epidemiological study using a health claims database to evaluate thyroid and other cancer risks as well as risks of hypoglycaemia, pancreatitis and allergic reactions; second, a cancer registry to evaluate the risk of medullary thyroid cancer over 15 years. Of note, no increase in calcitonin has been observed in clinical trials. Routine measurements of calcitonin are not required.

4.2.3 Administration and dosing

Liraglutide is formulated as a solution for subcutaneous injection in pre-filled pens delivering 0.6, 1.2 or 1.8 mg per dose. The suggested starting dose is 0.6 mg a day, increasing after not less than a week to a maintenance dose of 1.2 mg a day. After at least another week, and based on clinical response, the dose can be increased to 1.8 mg. In 2010, the National Institute for Health and Clinical Excellence (NICE) guidance recommended liraglutide (0.6 or 1.2 mg daily) as an option within a triple therapy regimen; the 1.8 mg dose was not recommended.

4.2.4 Efficacy and tolerability

In obese patients with type 2 diabetes liraglutide significantly lowers HbA_{1c} values and improves both fasting and postprandial glucose levels while reducing mean body weight 1–3 kg in a dose-dependent effect. The main adverse events with liraglutide are gastrointestinal, i.e. diarrhoea and nausea, although the frequency of these side-effects decreases over time. Liraglutide is associated with positive effects on cardiovascular biomarkers including the lowering of triglycerides and reductions in blood pressure. Islet β-cell function glucose sensitivity is increased, with enhanced potentiation of meal-associated insulin secretion. Postprandial glucagon levels are decreased. Liraglutide has not been studied in patients with severely impaired renal function and its use is not recommended for patients with moderate degrees of renal impairment, i.e. creatinine clearance of approximately 30–60 ml/min. Data in patients with hepatic impairment are limited.

A programme of phase III studies, the LEAD (Liraglutide Effect and Action in Diabetes) 1 to 6, demonstrated the efficacy of liraglutide as monotherapy, as add-on therapy to metformin or a sulphonylurea, and in combination with metformin, a sulphonylurea, or rosiglitazone. In the LEAD 6 study the efficacy and safety of liraglutide 1.8 mg once a day was compared with exenatide 10 μg twice a day in patients with inadequately controlled type 2 diabetes on maximally tolerated doses of metformin, sulphonylureas, or both. The mean baseline HbA_{1c} for the study population was approximately 8%. Liraglutide was associated with a significant reduction of approximately 0.3 percentage points in HbA_{1c} (Figure 3.4), and was generally better tolerated than exenatide. Nausea was less persistent with liraglutide, the percentages of patients affected being less than 5% compared with less than 10%, respectively, at 26 weeks. Both drugs promoted similar weight loss of approximately

3 kg. The incidence of minor hypoglycaemia was lower with liraglutide. Measures of β-cell function improved more with liraglutide. Decreases in fasting glucagon concentration and blood pressure were similar between the treatment groups, whereas fatty acids and triglycerides were reduced to a greater extent with liraglutide. Two patients taking exenatide together with a sulphonylurea had an episode of major hypoglycaemia, underscoring the need for caution when GLP-1 receptor agonists are combined with an insulin secretagogue. In the UK, the combination of GLP-1 receptor agonists or DPP-4 inhibitors with a sulphonylurea is regarded as being a potentially high-risk treatment for drivers holding group 2 (large goods and passenger carrying vehicles) licences; individual assessment is required (www.dvla.org.uk). The use of exenatide, liraglutide or a DPP-4 inhibitor currently carries no specific driving restrictions for group 1 (car or motorcycle) licences.

In preclinical studies thyroid C-cell tumours were observed in rats and mice. In 1% or fewer liraglutide-treated patients increased rates of thyroid-related adverse events have been observed, including neoplasms, elevated blood calcitonin levels and goitre. Anti-liraglutide antibody formation has been reported in less than 10% of patients, but these have not been associated with the decreased efficacy of the drug. A small number of cases of acute pancreatitis have been reported, but no clear evidence of causality has emerged. The utility of liraglutide for use as a weight-reducing drug in obese individuals without diabetes is under investigation.

5. Amylin analogues

Amylin, islet amyloid polypeptide, is a 37 residue peptide hormone that is co-secreted with insulin from islet β cells in response to meals. In humans, amylin

---

Figure 3.4. LEAD (Liraglutide Effect and Action in Diabetes) 6 study. Comparison of liraglutide 1.8 mg daily with exenatide 10 μg twice a day. Change in HbA$_{1c}$ from baseline after 26 weeks of treatment.

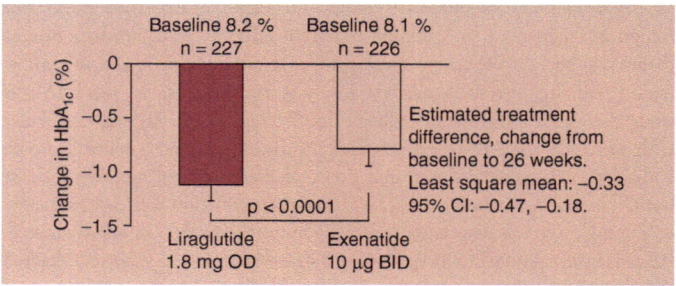

BID = Twice a day; HbA$_{1c}$ = glycated haemoglobin; OD = once a day.
Reproduced with permission from Buse et al. (2009).

precipitates and aggregates forming amyloid fibres, which play a putative role in the progressive β-cell destruction that characterises type 2 diabetes. The circulating hormone activates central neural pathways that decrease glucagon release from pancreatic α cells, retard gastric emptying and promote satiety.

5.1 Pramlintide

Pramlintide is a soluble synthetic amylin analogue that does not pre-cipitate. The drug exhibits similar pharmacokinetic and pharmacodynamic properties to native amylin. In the USA amylin is approved as adjunctive treatment in patients with type 2 diabetes using mealtime insulin, with or without the concurrent use of metformin and/or a sulphonylurea. It can also be used in patients with type 1 diabetes. The drug is not available in the UK. Studies of 4–52 weeks' duration examining the effect of pre-meal pramlintide injection in patients with type 2 diabetes have noted a re-duction in HbA_{1c} of approximately 0.5%. Two-hour postprandial glucose concentrations were reduced by nearly 3.5 mmol. The principal adverse effects of pramlintide are nausea and hypoglycaemia, the latter being two to fourfold higher than placebo during the first 4 weeks of therapy. Pramlintide is administered by subcutaneous injection; as a result of pH differences it must be given as a separate injection to insulin. The pre-meal dose of insulin may need to be reduced when pramlintide is initiated; the close self-monitoring of blood glucose concentrations is required. The delay in gastric emptying may mean that the administration of preprandial insulin may have to be delayed with the aim of matching peak insulin concentration with the rise in blood glucose. In patients with type 2 dia-betes treatment can be initiated at a dose of 60 µg (10 U) a day injected immediately before the main meal, titrated up to 120 µg. To reduce nausea, which usually subsides, the starting dose may be reduced to 30 µg (5 U) and the dose gradually increased according to tolerability. Weight loss of approximately 1–2 kg was sustained for 2 years or longer in open extension studies. In turn, weight reduction may help facilitate the long-term down-titration of insulin doses. This scenario contrasts with the common clinical situation in which the initiation of insulin therapy in the obese patient with type 2 diabetes results in further weight gain that ne-cessitates escalating insulin requirements. When combined with a sul-phonylurea, pramlintide may increase the risk of hypoglycaemia.

6. Bromocriptine

In 2009 a quick release (QR) formulation of the ergot alkaloid dopamine D2 receptor agonist bromocriptine was approved by the FDA for the treatment of type 2 diabetes as an adjunct to diet and exercise. Bromo-criptine-QR represents a novel application for a drug that has a well-established place in the treatment of hyperprolactinaemia and Parkinson's

> ## Box 3.1: Examples of novel glucose-lowering drugs reported to be in development for the treatment of type 2 diabetes
>
> **Class (phase of development)**
> - *Sodium-glucose co-transporter type 2 (SGLT2) inhibitors (II and III)*
> - *Immune modulators (III)*
> - *Incretin-based therapies (II and III)*
>   - *Dipeptidyl peptidase 4 (DPP-4) inhibitors*
>   - *Glucagon-like peptide 1 (GLP-1) receptor agonists*
> - *Peroxisome proliferator-activated receptor (PPAR) modulators (III)*
> - *Selective peroxisome proliferator-activated receptor γ modulators (SPPARMS) (II and III)*
> - *Sulphonylurea receptor modulators (III)*
> - *Glucokinase activators (I and II)*
> - *G protein-coupled receptor 119 (GPR119) agonists (I)*
> - *Glucocorticoid pathway modulators (IIb)*
> - *Ultra-long-acting insulin analogues (III) (see chapter 2)*
> - *Novel insulin formulations (II and III)*
>   - *Inhaled insulin*
>   - *Oral insulin*

disease. It is postulated that by providing a short duration central dopaminergic pulse, bromocriptine-QR enhances insulin sensitivity and improves aspects of endocrine function and intermediary metabolism thereby reducing cardiovascular risk. In clinical trials, as monotherapy or in combination with other glucose-lowering drugs, bromocriptine-QR lowered glycated haemoglobin by 0.6–1.2%. The drug is taken with food within 2 h of waking in order to coincide with the physiological peak in dopaminergic tone. The initial dose is one tablet (0.8 mg) daily, increased weekly by one tablet until a maximal tolerated daily dose of 1.6–4.8 mg is attained. The main dose-limiting side-effect is nausea. In accordance with FDA requirements, a 52-week safety trial was conducted in 3095 patients. This reported a statistically significant 40% lower incidence of cardiovascular events in bromocriptine-QR-treated subjects compared with placebo.

7. Drugs in development

Several classes of novel drugs with glucose-reducing properties are in development for type 2 diabetes (Box 3.1). Recent safety concerns about thiazolidinediones and theoretical reservations about new drugs acting on the incretin axis have heightened awareness of the need for rigorous evaluation of new therapies. Whether examples from the classes discussed here will ultimately be approved rests on the results of clinical trials. As discussed in Chapter 1, the FDA has signalled the need for rigorous assessment of the cardiovascular risks of novel glucose-lowering agents. Of the oral agents currently in phase III clinical trials sodium-glucose co-transporter type 2 inhibitors are attracting the greatest attention. These drugs reduce the renal tubular reabsorption of glucose thereby reducing hyperglycaemia. Increased urinary calorie excretion promotes weight loss. The risk of hypoglycaemia is low. Reductions in blood pressure have been reported. The frequency of urogenital infections is increased. Intravascular volume depletion is a potential side-effect that might be deleterious in patients with compromised renal function. Dapagliflozin has led the field in this class of new agents while others, including canagliflozin, are in various stages of development. An imbalance of cancer of the bladder and breast was observed in phase III studies of dapagliflozin. To date, no mechanistic basis for the latter observation has been identified. In July 2011 an FDA advisory committee declined approval for dapagliflozin. Renal and liver safety concerns, especially in the elderly, were also raised.

In January 2012 the FDA rejected approval for dapagliflozin pending submission of more data on benefits and safety. In April 2012, the Committee for Medicinal Products for Human Use (CHMP) of the EMA recommended the approval of dapagliflozin for the treatment of type 2 diabetes as an adjunct to diet and exercise, in combination with other glucose-lowering drugs including insulin, and as a monotherapy in metformin intolerant patients.

Ultra-long insulin analogues are under development. The potential advantages of this approach are considered in Chapter 2.

Further reading

Bray GA. Lifestyle and pharmacological approaches to weight loss: efficacy and safety. *J Clin Endocrinol Metab.* 2008;93(Suppl. 1):S81-8.

Buse JB, Rosenstock J, Sesti G, et al. Liraglutide once a day versus exenatide twice a day for type 2 diabetes: a 26-week randomised, parallel-group, multinational, open-label trial (LEAD-6). *Lancet.* 2009;374:39-47.

Defronzo RA. Bromocriptine: a sympatholytic, d2-dopamine agonist for the treatment of type 2 diabetes. *Diabetes Care.* 2011;34:789-94.

Drucker DJ, Buse JB, Taylor K, et al. DURATION-1 Study Group. Exenatide once weekly versus twice daily for the treatment of type 2 diabetes: a randomised, open-label, non-inferiority study. *Lancet.* 2008;372:1240-50.

Drucker DJ, Nauck MA. The incretin system: glucagon-like peptide-1 receptor agonists and dipeptidyl peptidase-4 inhibitors in type 2 diabetes. *Lancet.* 2006;368:1696-705.

Flatt PR, Bailey CJ, Green BD. Recent advances in antidiabetic drug therapies targeting the enteroinsular axis. *Curr Drug Metab.* 2009;10:125-37.

Gallwitz B, Häring HU. Future perspectives for insulinotropic agents in the treatment of type 2 diabetes – DPP-4 inhibitors and sulphonylureas. *Diabetes Obes Metab.* 2010;12:1-11.

Gerich JE. Role of the kidney in normal glucose homeostasis and in the hyperglycaemia of diabetes mellitus: therapeutic implications. *Diabetic Med.* 2010;27:136-42.

Hanefeld M, Forst T. Dapagliflozin, an SGLT2 inhibitor, for diabetes. *Lancet.* 2010;375:2196-8.

Henry RR, Lincoff AM, Mudaliar S, et al. Effect of the dual peroxisome proliferator-activated receptor-alpha/gamma agonist aleglitazar on risk of cardiovascular disease in patients with type 2 diabetes (SYNCHRONY): a phase II, randomised, dose-ranging study. *Lancet.* 2009;374:126-35.

Hoogwerf BJ, Doshi KB, Diab D. Pramlintide, the synthetic analogue of amylin: physiology, pathophysiology, and effects on glycemic control, body weight, and selected biomarkers of vascular risk. *Vasc Health Risk Manage.* 2008;4:355-62.

Idris I, Donnelly R. Sodium-glucose co-transporter-2 inhibitors: an emerging new class of oral antidiabetic drug. *Diabetes Obes Metab.* 2009;11:79-88.

Krentz AJ. New oral agents for type 2 diabetes. *Clin Med* 2007;7:117-8.

Krentz AJ, Patel M, Bailey CJ. New therapies for type 2 diabetes – what is their place in therapy? *Drugs.* 2008;68:2131-62.

Nauck M, Stöckmann F, Ebert R, Creutzfeldt W. Reduced incretin effect in type 2 (non-insulin-dependent) diabetes. *Diabetologia* 1986;29:46-52.

National Institute for Health and Clinical Excellence. Type 2 diabetes. *Clinical guideline 87.* May 2009. Available at: www.nice.org.uk/nicemedia/pdf/CG87NICEGuideline.pdf. Accessed 2010 Apr 19

Norris SL, Lee N, Thakurta S, Chan BK. Exenatide efficacy and safety: a systematic review. *Diabet Med.* 2009;26:837-46.

Richter B, Bandeira-Echtler E, Bergerhoff K, Lerch CL. Dipeptidyl peptidase-4 (DPP-4) inhibitors for type 2 diabetes mellitus. *Cochrane Database Sys Rev.* 2008;Issue 2. Art. No.: CD006739.

Todd JF, Bloom SR. Incretins and other peptides in the treatment of diabetes. *Diabet Med.* 2007;24:223-32.

Chapter 4

The place of newer drugs in treatment algorithms

1. Recommended management of type 2 diabetes

Several national and international guidelines have been published for the treatment of type 2 diabetes. These partially duplicate one another and no single guideline has been universally adopted. Factors that should be taken into consideration when reviewing the options include: whether a consensus panel versus a structured evidence-based approach was used; the importance of drug costs and issues of cost-effectiveness; the enthusiasm for newer versus more established agents; known and as yet uncertain short and longer-term safety issues.

In 2009, guidance was issued by the National Institute for Health and Clinical Excellence (NICE) for some newer glucose-lowering agents that partly updated earlier guidelines.

1. The dipeptidyl peptidase 4 (DPP-4) inhibitors, sitagliptin and vildagliptin; saxagliptin had not be approved at this time.
2. The thiazolidinediones, pioglitazone and rosiglitazone – including new data on cardiovascular safety and clinical effectiveness.
3. The glucagon-like peptide 1 (GLP-1) mimetic exenatide; liraglutide was not available.
4. The prolonged duration insulin analogues, insulin glargine and insulin detemir.

NICE is an independent organisation responsible for providing national guidance on the promotion of good health and the prevention and treatment of ill health in England and Wales. Scotland has separate evidence-based guidelines published by the Scottish Intercollegiate Guidelines Network (SIGN). NICE assesses the cost-effectiveness of new therapies. This involves an analysis of the cost and benefit of proposed treatment relative to current therapy using quality-adjusted life-years (QALY) to assess health benefits. The influence of NICE increasingly extends beyond the UK. NICE provides an evidence-based assessment of treatment options for the National Health Service (NHS). Other guidelines for the management of type 2 diabetes that are widely quoted at international level include the American Diabetes Association (ADA)/European Association for the Study of Diabetes (EASD) guidance, which has been presented as a consensus statement, and the more evidence-based International Diabetes Federation (IDF) global guidelines. The latter offers three standards of care – comprehensive, standard and minimal in recognition of global variations in healthcare provision for diabetes.

A. J. Krentz, *Drug Therapy for Type 2 Diabetes*,
DOI: 10.1007/978-1-908517-77-7_4,
© Springer International Publishing Switzerland 2012

The recommendations of the American Association of Clinical Endocrinologists (AACE)/American College of Endocrinology (ACE) and those of the Canadian Diabetes Association (CDA) also attract attention beyond their national boundaries.

There has been a move in guideline development towards the use of more systematic literature reviews; wider consultation with representatives of professional bodies and patient advocacy groups are in favour. Rather than emphasising minor differences between the leading guidelines, attention might more usefully be drawn to the practical difficulties that attend their implementation, e.g. clinical inertia and local budgetary constraints. The IDF provides detailed instructions for the development of national guidelines. Many countries have indeed established their own national guidelines to reflect issues such as particular local needs and government drug reimbursement policies.

2. Current NICE guidance: oral glucose-lowering drugs

This guidance is based on detailed consideration of current evidence. In the NHS, NICE requires healthcare professionals to take the guidance into account when exercising clinical judgement. The guidance is not, however, intended to override the responsibility of healthcare professionals to make decisions appropriate to the circumstances of the individual patient. This should be done in consultation with the patient and/or their guardian or carer, and informed by the current summary of the product characteristics of specific drugs. Other important points about the scope and rationale of the guidance is presented in Box 4.1.

Box 4.1: NICE guidance 87

This 2009 clinical guideline covers newer agents for blood glucose control in adults with type 2 diabetes and is a partial update of Type 2 Diabetes, NICE clinical guideline 66, published in 2008.

- *The guideline addresses only the licensed use of drugs.*
- *The guidance does not address care for pregnant women with diabetes.*
- *Exenatide is licensed as a drug to lower blood glucose in diabetes and not as a drug to promote weight loss.*
- *The use of prolonged duration insulin analogues is considered only in comparison with neutral protamine Hagedorn (NPH) insulin.*
- *Levels of glycated haemoglobin (HbA_{1c}) that should prompt consideration of additional glucose-lowering agents are: (a) >6.5% for people on one glucose-lowering drug and (b) ≥7.5% for people on two or more oral glucose-lowering drugs, or individuals needing insulin. These different levels take into account the increasing risk of hypoglycaemia with insulin and the clinical and cost-effectiveness of newer agents.*

Figure 4.1. Care pathway for type 2 diabetes. NICE guidance 87 (2009).

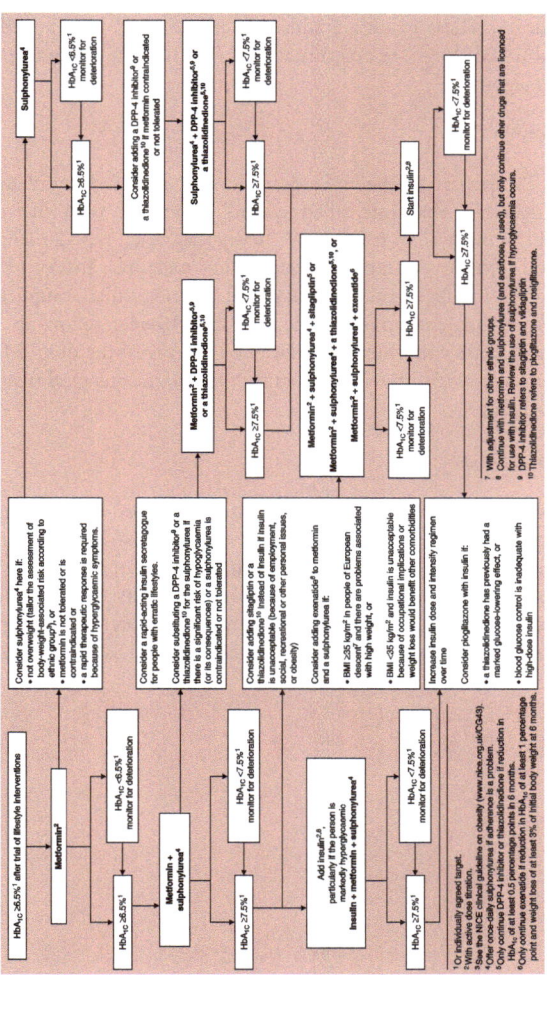

BMI = Body mass index; DPP-4 = dipeptidyl peptidase 4; HbA₁c = glycated haemoglobin.

Adapted from National Institute for Health and Clinical Excellence (2009), with permission.

NICE guidance (Figure 4.1) sets the management of type 2 diabetes within a framework of patient-centred care (Box 4.2). Treatment and care should take into account the needs and preferences of the patient. Inevitably, national guidelines require periodic updates to accommodate the arrival of new agents and changes in approval or safety warnings for existing drugs. These issues are addressed in the latest NICE guidance. Well-established drugs are accommodated within a revised and updated treatment algorithm.

2.1 Metformin

The UK Prospective Diabetes Study (UKPDS) provided key data supporting the view that intensified control compared with diet using metformin in overweight people with newly diagnosed type 2 diabetes is logical and effective. Compared with dietary measures, metformin was associated with reduced microvascular and macrovascular complications and improved patient survival. The post-trial 10-year follow-up study published in 2008 confirmed the continued efficacy of the drug. Metformin therefore provides the foundation for oral pharmacological treatment of type 2 diabetes.

2.2 Sulphonylureas

Sulphonylureas continue to be widely used. For non-obese patients a sulphonylurea may be considered as an alternative first-line treatment to metformin. Prescribing a sulphonylurea with metformin remains the most common combination of oral glucose-lowering agents. If, however, the avoidance of hypoglycaemia is particularly important, e.g. for patients whose occupations are potentially hazardous or in frail elderly individuals,

---

Box 4.2: Patient-centred care: NICE guidelines

- *Treatment and care should take into account patients' needs and preferences.*
- *People with type 2 diabetes should be able to make informed decisions about their care and treatment, in partnership with healthcare professionals.*
- *Good communication between healthcare professionals and patients is essential and should be supported by evidence-based written information tailored to the needs of the patient.*
- *Treatment and care, and the information patients are given about it, should be culturally appropriate and tailored to individual circumstances.*
- *With the patient's agreement, families and carers should have the opportunity to be involved in decisions about treatment and care.*
- *Families and carers should also be given the information and support they need.*

then a thiazolidinedione or a DPP-4 inhibitor may be added to metformin as an alternative to a sulphonylurea.

2.3 Prandial glucose regulators

The short-acting prandial glucose regulators, repaglinide and nateglinide, are not regarded as having significant advantages over other insulin secretagogues. However, the risk of hypoglycaemia may be lower with these agents than for sulphonylureas; this may be of value in older patients, particularly in the presence of renal impairment. These drugs may play a useful role in patients with unpredictable lifestyles. Flexibility may be granted using these agents if strictly timed main meals are problematic, as these agents are taken immediately before eating. If a meal is missed, the appropriate dose of repaglinide is omitted. The use of these drugs in the UK has been very limited.

2.4 Thiazolidinediones

Pioglitazone is approved for use as monotherapy, or in combination with metformin or a sulphonylurea. The drug may be used in combination with both metformin and a sulphonylurea. Pioglitazone is also approved for use in combination with insulin. Clinical trial data indicate that pioglitazone is a potential alternative option to adding basal insulin to a metformin–sulphonylurea combination; however, an eventual need for insulin replacement therapy should be anticipated as β-cell function wanes. The pros and cons of using pioglitazone in favour of adding insulin should be carefully considered; an informed choice should be made by the patient. Cultural considerations may be relevant when insulin therapy is being offered. The NICE guidelines and the ADA/EASD consensus statement recommend that a sulphonylurea be used as preferred second-line therapy when metformin monotherapy brings insufficient control of hyperglycaemia. The use of pioglitazone as second-line therapy should be considered if the person is at significant risk of hypoglycaemia or if a sulphonylurea is not tolerated or is contraindicated. It is important to remember that 6–8 weeks or more may be required for the maximal glucose-lowering effect of pioglitazone to be achieved. If the glycated haemoglobin (HbA_{1c}) level has not been lowered at least 0.5% by 6 months the thiazolidinedione should be discontinued. NICE stipulates that pioglitazone should not be initiated or continued in patients who have heart failure, or are predisposed to skeletal fractures.

2.5 Acarbose

Acarbose is regarded as being generally less effective than metformin and sulphonylureas. It can be used as monotherapy or in combination with other agents. However, the high incidence of gastrointestinal side effects has been a major barrier to its use, at least in the UK. Miglitol is not available.

2.6 Dipeptidyl peptidase-4 inhibitors

DPP-4 inhibitors can be used in combination with metformin, a sulphonylurea or a thiazolidinedione. Sitagliptin has EMA approval for restricted use as monotherapy when metformin is contraindicated. The use of sitagliptin in combination with metformin together with a sulphonylurea is approved. In 2009, the use of sitagliptin as an adjunct to insulin therapy was approved. The NICE guidelines recommend that when glycaemic control remains or becomes inadequate, i.e. HbA_{1c} is 6.5% or more or another level agreed with the patient, and hypoglycaemia is a concern, a DPP-4 inhibitor may be considered in place of a sulphonylurea as second-line treatment with metformin. If metformin is not tolerated or is contraindicated, a DPP-4 inhibitor may be added to a sulphonylurea. This option may be preferable to adding a thiazolidinedione if avoidance of weight gain or intolerance are concerns. A DPP-4 inhibitor should only be continued if a satisfactory glycaemic response, defined as a reduction in HbA_{1c} of at least 0.5%, is achieved by 6 months.

3. NICE guidance: injectable agents

3.1 Glucagon-like peptide-1 agonists: exenatide and liraglutide

The 2009 NICE guidance recommends that the GLP-1 agonist exenatide be considered as third-line therapy (if HbA_{1c} is ≥7.5%) added to metformin in conjunction with a sulphonylurea when the body mass index (BMI) is $35.0 \, kg/m^2$ or greater with associated psychological or medical problems, or the BMI is less than $35.0 \, kg/m^2$ but insulin therapy would have substantial occupational implications or weight loss would benefit serious obesity-associated co-morbidities. Note that a lower BMI threshold is appropriate for patients of non-European ethnicity. Exenatide should only be continued if a beneficial response is observed, defined as a reduction of at least 1.0 percentage point in HbA_{1c} and a weight loss of at least 3% of initial body weight at 6 months. The stipulation of a dual response for glycaemic control and weight, if rigidly adhered to, could deny benefits for patients with serious co-morbidities. For example, patients with obesity-associated obstructive sleep apnoea might not reach the target for HbA_{1c} reduction while achieving clinically important weight loss.

Since publication of the 2009 NICE guidance liraglutide has become available in the UK. NICE guidance issued in 2010 recommends use of liraglutide as part of triple therapy with oral therapies at a maximum daily dose of 1.2 mg. Body weight stipulations are similar to those applicable for exenatide.

3.2 Insulin glargine and insulin detemir

In addition to providing recommendations for the six available classes of oral glucose-lowering drugs and the only GLP-1 agonist available at the time, the 2009 NICE guidelines considered the place of the prolonged duration insulin analogues insulin detemir and insulin glargine. These have been available for several years and are widely used in the UK. In brief, and in contrast to the latest AACE/ACE guidance, NICE continues to recommend NPH (neutral protamine Hagedorn) insulin when insulin therapy is commenced in patients with type 2 diabetes. NICE acknowledges a role for insulin analogues, the main advantages of insulin glargine and insulin detemir over NPH being a lower risk of hypoglycaemia at comparable degrees of glucose control and a lesser effect on body weight. The NICE guidance provides advice on the initiation and adjustment of insulin therapy in patients with type 2 diabetes (Box 4.3) A detailed algorithm is also offered in the ADA/EASD guidelines.

4. National and international guidelines compared

While similarities dominate, there are some differences in approach between current guidelines. Many of these are minor. More notable differences in clinical practice are, however, also evident between expert groups. The 2006 and 2009 ADA/EASD guidance classified drugs by whether or not they were deemed well-validated (Figure 4.2). This reflects the history of accumulated clinical experience with different classes – and individual agents within classes – and outcome data from major clinical trials. This model provides the basis for a stepwise approach to treatment. By definition, all newer agents such as DPP-4 inhibitors and GLP-1 agonists cannot be categorised as well-validated core therapy and so are viewed as being alternatives to metformin, sulphonylureas and insulin. Consideration was also given to metabolic effects other than glucose lowering, e.g. changes in lipid profiles. GLP-1 agonists and pioglitazone are listed as less well-validated tier 2 therapies. An updated 2012 ADA/EASD position statement abandoned selection of drugs by validation in favour of a more flexible patient-centred and individualized approach.

The inclusion of therapeutic efficacy targets for newer agents in the NICE guidelines may reduce needless expense incurred by the futile use of high-cost newer agents when more appropriate action should be taken, e.g. a timely move to insulin therapy. The stipulations of a reduction in HbA_{1c} of 0.5% or greater after 6 months of therapy for a DPP-4 inhibitor and 1.0% for exenatide are broadly in line with responses reported in clinical trials.

Box 4.3: Summary of insulin initiation, monitoring, and intensification of therapy in patients with type 2 diabetes

From NICE Guidance 87 (2009)

- *Begin with human neutral protamine Hagedorn (NPH) insulin injected at bedtime or twice daily according to need.*

- *Consider, as an alternative, initiating insulin therapy using a long-acting insulin analogue (insulin detemir, insulin glargine) if the patient:*

  - *needs assistance from a carer or healthcare professional to inject insulin, and the use of a long-acting insulin analogue (insulin detemir, insulin glargine) would reduce the frequency of injections from twice to once daily, or*

  - *has their lifestyle restricted by recurrent symptomatic hypoglycaemic episodes, or*

  - *would otherwise need twice-daily NPH insulin injections in combination with oral glucose-lowering drugs, or*

  - *cannot use the device to inject NPH insulin.*

- *Consider twice-daily pre-mixed (biphasic) human insulin (particularly if glycated haemoglobin [HbA_{1c}] ≥9.0%). A once-daily regimen is an alternative option.*

- *Consider pre-mixed preparations that include short-acting insulin analogues, rather than pre-mixed preparations that include short-acting human insulin preparations, if:*

  - *the patient prefers injecting insulin immediately before a meal, or*

  - *hypoglycaemia is a problem, or*

  - *blood glucose levels rise markedly after meals.*

- *Consider switching to a prolonged duration insulin analogue (insulin detemir, insulin glargine) from NPH insulin in people:*

  - *who do not reach their target HbA_{1c} because of significant hypoglycaemia, or*

  - *who experience significant hypoglycaemia on NPH insulin irrespective of the level of HbA_{1c} reached, or*

  - *who cannot use the device needed to inject NPH insulin but who could administer their own insulin safely and accurately if a switch to a long-acting insulin analogue was made, or*

  - *who need help from a carer or healthcare professional to administer insulin injections and for whom switching to a long-acting insulin analogue would reduce the number of daily injections.*

- *Monitor a person on a basal insulin regimen (for the need for short-acting insulin before meals or a pre-mixed insulin preparation).*

- *Monitor a person who is using pre-mixed insulin once or twice daily for the need for a further injection of short-acting insulin before meals or for a change to a regimen of mealtime plus basal insulin, if blood glucose control remains inadequate.*

Figure 4.2. Algorithm for the metabolic management of hyperglycaemia in type 2 diabetes. Reinforce lifestyle interventions at every visit and check glycated haemoglobin (HbA$_{1c}$) every 3 months until HbA$_{1c}$ is <7% and then at least every 6 months. The interventions should be changed if HbA$_{1c}$ is ≥7%.

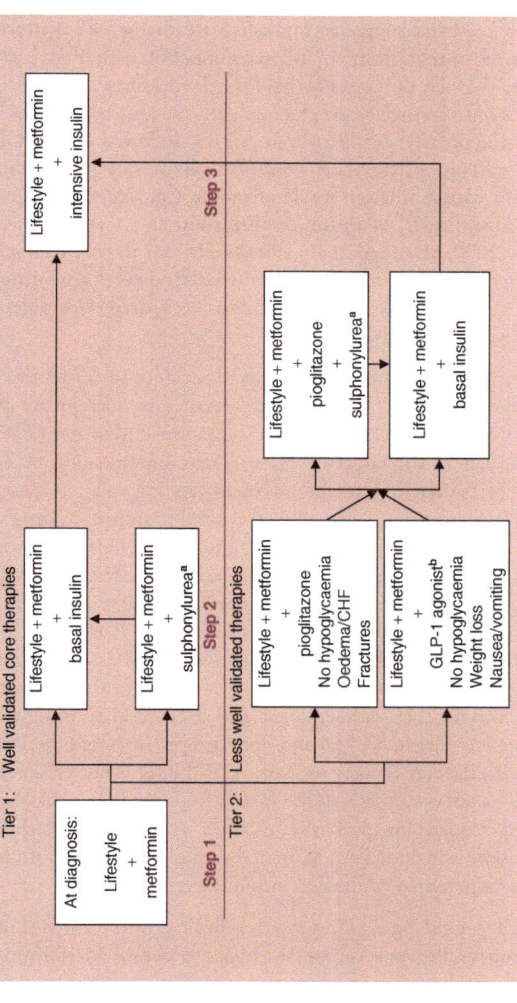

[a]Sulphonylureas other than glybenclamide (glyburide) or chlorpropamide.

[b]Insufficient clinical use to be confident regarding safety.

CHF = Congestive heart failure; GLP-1 = glucagon-like peptide 1.

Adapted from Nathan et al. (2009), with permission.

Combination drug therapy is needed for the majority of patients, and increasingly the view is taken that this should be considered at an early stage. In the UK metformin is the drug of choice with which to initiate pharmacotherapy. The NICE and ADA/EASD guidelines differ in their recommendations about when metformin should be started. The 2009 ADA/EASD guideline suggested immediate treatment with metformin, in the absence of contraindications and in conjunction with lifestyle changes. This reflects the view of the panel that lifestyle measures alone are unlikely to be sufficient to control blood glucose levels. In contrast, NICE suggests a sequential approach, i.e. lifestyle measures, followed by metformin if indicated and appropriate. This would be followed by the addition of a second agent with a different mode of action, e.g. a sulphonylurea, or in the 2009 ADA/EASD algorithm, with insulin as a well-validated alternative. The 2009 ADA/EASD guidelines called for the preferential use of second-generation sulphonylureas and their extended release formulations in view of the lower risk of hypoglycaemia compared with older agents such as glibenclamide (glyburide).

The AACE/ACE guidelines stratify the choice of initial therapy by HbA_{1c}. These guidelines advocate the use of dual therapy for patients with an HbA_{1c} of 7.5% to 9% using the rationale that monotherapy is unlikely to achieve the target of 6.5%. Triple combination therapy (or insulin if the patient has symptoms of hyperglycaemia), is a suggested option if HbA_{1c} is greater than 9.0%. Several examples of drug combinations are offered in the AACE/ACE guidelines. This approach is reflected in the prioritisation of therapy according to safety – especially the risk of hypoglycaemia – and glucose-lowering efficacy, as well as judgements about predicted adherence to therapy. Cost is regarded as a secondary consideration. DPP-4 inhibitors are regarded as suitable first-line therapy, along with other drugs that carry a negligible risk of hypogycaemia – metformin, thiazolidinediones, and α-glucosidase inhibitors; sulphonylureas are relegated to second-line therapy. It should be noted that gliclazide MR, the core therapy used in ADVANCE, is not available in the USA and so is not considered in the AACE/ACE guidelines. Colesevelam, a bile acid sequestrant primarily used to reduce plasma cholesterol concentrations, is included as a potential second-line drug. Pramlintide is suggested as a potential adjunct to insulin therapy.

The CDA guidelines places metformin first, in the absence of metabolic decompensation or symptomatic hyperglycaemia. Metformin should be initiated simultaneously with nutrition therapy and increased physical activity – with or without an agent from a different class – if HbA_{1c} is greater than 9.0%. Thereafter, if glycaemic targets are not achieved another agent, which may be a weight-reducing drug, should be added as best suited to the individual. Some key points from the IDF and CDA guidelines are presented in Box 4.4. The 2005 IDF guideline did not include drugs such as DPP-4 inhibitors. An algorithm published in 2011 updated the guidance to include newer therapies (www.idf.org/treatment-algorithm-people-type-2-diabetes). This was followed in 2012 by an updated guideline (www.idf.org/global-guideline-type-2-diabetes-2012). This includes the options offered by newer classes of newer glucose-lowering drugs including agents acting on the incretin axis. A step-wise approach is recommended which commences with metformin. Sulphonylureas are the preferred second-line option. The generic algorithm is offered with the expectation that individual countries will modify the details according to availability, access and medication costs. Attention is drawn to higher price of proprietary drugs compared with generic versions and newer versus older drugs. Such considerations are of particular relevance to middle and low-income countries.

The NICE guidelines set an optimal target of 6.5% for HbA_{1c}, whereas the ADA/EASD target is 7.0%. It is re-emphasised that targets should be set according to individual characteristics and in collaboration with the patient. The IDF target is less than 6.5%, with equivalent target

---

Box 4.4: Key points from the 2005 International Diabetes Federation (IDF) and the 2008 Canadian Diabetes Association guidelines for glucose-lowering therapies. The IDF guideline was updated in 2012 to include DPP-4 inhibitors and GLP-1 receptor agonists.

International Diabetes Federation (IDF)[*]

- *Start metformin after lifestyle interventions; a sulphonylurea or pioglitazone*[†] *as alternatives.*
- *Move to metformin plus sulphonylurea. Choose low-cost sulphonylureas but consider once daily formulation if concordance is problematical.*
- *Then add pioglitazone*[†] *or acarbose to metformin plus sulphonylurea.*
- *Start insulin; intensify as necessary.*

Canadian Diabetes Association

- *Metformin first, in the absence of metabolic decompensation or symptomatic hyperglycaemia.*
- *Metformin initiated simultaneously with nutrition therapy and increased physical activity – with or without an agent from a different class – if HbA_{1c} is greater than 9.0%.*
- *If glycaemic targets are not achieved, another agent, including weight-loss drugs, should be added as best suited to the individual.*

[*] *The IDF has also published a separate guideline on the management of postprandial hyperglycaemia.*
[†] *Rosiglitazone withdrawn in 2010.*

levels for capillary plasma glucose levels of less than 6.0 mmol/l before meals and less than 8.0 mmol/l 1–2 h after meals. In general, and based on a consideration of the somewhat conflicting results of the ACCORD (Action to Control Cardiovascular Risk in Diabetes), ADVANCE (Action in Diabetes and Vascular Disease: Preterax and Diamicron Modified Release Controlled Evaluation) and the VADT (Veterans Affairs Diabetes Trial), patients with known duration diabetes of less than a decade with no evidence of cardiovascular disease should aim for an HbA$_{1c}$ level of 7.0% or less. If a lower level can safely be achieved without compromising quality of life, ideally by non-pharmacological means, this would be expected to bring additional long-term protection against the development and progression of microangiopathy, as reported in ADVANCE. The results of the latter study have, however, not prompted a revision of the ADA target for HbA$_{1c}$. The question of whether intensive blood glucose control will lead to a significant reduction in macrovascular events is not answered by the aforementioned trials, none of which was of sufficient duration to address the hypothesis reliably. The importance of the overall therapeutic strategy should be kept in mind when selecting glucose-lowering pharmacotherapy. Recent clinical trials provide support for a measured escalation of drug therapy. The intensive use of combinations of drugs from different classes may increase the risk of severe hypoglycaemia and excessive weight gain. As ever, the challenge for clinicians lies in weighing the predicted benefits against potential risks in the context of the needs of the individual.

Further reading

Canadian Diabetes Association. 2008 Clinical practice guidelines for the prevention and management of diabetes in Canada. *Can J Diabetes*. 2008;32(Suppl. 1):S1-201.

International Diabetes Federation. Clinical Guidelines Task Force. *Guide for guidelines. A guide for clinical guideline development.* 2003. Available at: www.idf.org.

International Diabetes Federation. Clinical Guidelines Task Force. *Global guideline for type 2 diabetes.* Brussels, 2005. Available at: www.idf.org.

Inzucchi SE, Bergenstal R, Buse JD, et al. Management of hyperglycemia in type 2 diabetes: a patient-centered approach. *Diabetes Care.* 2012;35:1364-79.

Kahn R, Gale EA. Gridlocked guidelines for diabetes.. *Lancet.* 2010;375:2203-4.

Krentz AJ, Bailey CJ. Oral antidiabetic agents: current role in type 2 diabetes mellitus. *Drugs.* 2005;65:385-411.

Nathan DM, Buse JB, Davidson MB, et al. Management of hyperglycaemia in type 2 diabetes mellitus: a consensus algorithm for the initiation and adjustment of therapy: a consensus statement from the American Diabetes Association and the European Association for the Study of Diabetes. *Diabetologia.* 2009;52:17-30.

National Collaborating Centre for Chronic Conditions. Type 2 diabetes: national clinical guideline for management in primary and secondary care (update). London: Royal College of Physicians, 2008.

National Institute for Health and Clinical Excellence. *The management of type 2 diabetes (update)*. (Clinical Guideline 66). London: NICE, 2008. Available at: www.nice.org.uk/CG66.

National Institute for Health and Clinical Excellence. *Type 2 diabetes: newer agents for blood glucose control in type 2 diabetes 2009*. (Clinical Guideline 87). London: NICE, 2009. Available at: www.nice.org.uk/CG87.

Rodbard HW, Jellinger PS, Davidson JA, et al. Statement by an American Association of Clinical Endocrinologists/American College of Endocrinology consensus panel on type 2 diabetes mellitus: an algorithm for glycemic control. *Endocr Pract.* 2009;15:540-59.

Sibal L, Home PD. Management of type 2 diabetes: NICE guidelines. *Clin Med.* 2009;9:353-7.

Stratton UM, Adler AI, Neil AW, et al. Association of glycaemia with macrovascular and microvascular complications of type 2 diabetes (UKPDS 35): prospective observational study. *BMJ.* 2000;321:405-12.

Index

A. J. Krentz, *Drug Therapy for Type 2 Diabetes*,
DOI: 10.1007/978-1-908517-77-7,
© Springer International Publishing Switzerland 2012